The Roles of Physician Assistants and Nurse Practitioners in Primary Care

D. Kay Clawson

Marian Osterweis

Editors

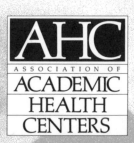

AHC

ASSOCIATION OF
ACADEMIC
HEALTH
CENTERS

T HE ASSOCIATION OF ACADEMIC HEALTH CENTERS (AHC) is a national, nonprofit organization comprising more than 100 institutional members in the United States and Canada that are the health complexes of the major universities of these nations. Academic health centers consist of an allopathic or osteopathic school of medicine, at least one other health professions school or program, and one or more teaching hospitals. These institutions are the primary resources for education in the health professions, biomedical and health services research, and many aspects of patient care services.

The AHC seeks to influence public dialogue on significant health and science policy issues, to advance education for health professionals, to promote biomedical and health services research, and to enhance patient care. The AHC is dedicated to improving the health of the people through leadership and cooperative action with others.

The preparation and publication of this book were supported by a grant from the Josiah Macy, Jr. Foundation.

The views expressed in this book are those of its authors and do not necessarily represent the views of the Board of Directors of the Association of Academic Health Centers or the membership at large.

ISBN 1-879694-07-7

Copies of this publication are available from:
Association of Academic Health Centers
1400 Sixteenth Street, N.W., Suite 410
Washington, D.C. 20036
202/265-9600 Fax: 202/265-7514

Design and Production: Fletcher Design, Washington, D.C.

Cover photo by Uniphoto, Washington, D.C./Pictor

This book is printed on recycled paper.

Contents

Contributors

James Cawley, P.A., M.P.H., is associate professor and director of the Physician Assistant Program at the George Washington University Medical Center in Washington, D.C.

D. Kay Clawson, M.D., is executive vice chancellor of the University of Kansas Medical Center in Kansas City, Kansas.

Henry Desmarais, M.D., M.P.A., is a principal with Health Policy Alternatives, Inc., in Washington, D.C.

E. Harvey Estes, Jr., M.D., is director of the Reynolds Community Practitioner Program for the North Carolina Medical Society Foundation in Raleigh, North Carolina.

Virginia Fowkes, M.H.S., is a senior research scholar and director of the Primary Care Associate Program in the division of family and community medicine in the School of Medicine at Stanford University in Palo Alto, California.

Stephen Garfinkel is a free-lance health writer in Washington, D.C.

Roderick S. Hooker, P.A., M.B.A., is adjunct investigator at the Center for Health Services Research and a clinician in the department of internal medicine of Kaiser Permanente Center for Health Research in Portland, Oregon.

Denis Oliver, Ph.D., is professor and director of the Physician Assistant Program at the University of Iowa in Iowa City, Iowa.

Marian Osterweis, Ph.D., is vice president and secretary and treasurer of the Association of Academic Health Centers.

Sheila Ryan, Ph.D., is dean of the School of Nursing and director of Medical Center Nursing at the University of Rochester Medical Center in Rochester, New York.

Barbara Starfield, M.D., M.P.H., is professor and head of the division of health policy in the School of Hygiene and Public Health at The Johns Hopkins University in Baltimore, Maryland.

ASSOCIATION OF ACADEMIC HEALTH CENTERS

The Roles of Physician Assistants and Nurse Practitioners in Primary Care

Workshop
Washington, D.C.   April 13, 1993
Participants

Task Force on Human Resources for Health

Paul F. Larson, M.D.
Senior Vice President for Academic
  Affairs
University of Medicine & Dentistry of
  New Jersey
Task Force Associate Chairman

Philip S. Birnbaum
Professor of Health Care Sciences
George Washington University
  Medical Center

Peter P. Bosomworth, M.D.
Chancellor for the Medical Center
University of Kentucky

D. Kay Clawson, M.D.
Executive Vice Chancellor
University of Kansas Medical Center
Task Force Chairman

James K. Hackett
Associate Vice President for
  Health Sciences
West Virginia University
Health Sciences Center

H. Garland Hershey, Jr., D.D.S.
Vice Chancellor for Health Affairs
  and
Vice Provost of the University
The University of North Carolina
  at Chapel Hill

James C. Hunt, M.D.
University Distinguished Professor
The University of Tennessee,
  Memphis

Elaine Larson, R.N., Ph.D.
Dean, School of Nursing
Georgetown University
*AHC Scholar in Academic
  Administration & Health Policy*

Henri R. Manasse, Jr., Ph.D.
Interim Vice Chancellor for Health
  Services
University of Illinois at Chicago

W. Marcus Newberry, Jr., M.D.
Vice President for Academic Affairs
  and Provost
Medical University of South Carolina

David J. Ramsay, D.M., D.Phil.
Senior Vice Chancellor/Academic
  Affairs
University of California,
  San Francisco

Harvey Sparks, M.D.
Vice Provost for Human Health
  Programs
Michigan State University

Ciro V. Sumaya, M.D., M.P.H.T.M.
Associate Dean for Affiliated
  Programs and Continuing Medical
  Education
The University of Texas Health
  Science Center at San Antonio
*AHC Scholar in Academic
  Administration & Health Policy*

Neal A. Vanselow, M.D.
Chancellor
Tulane University Medical Center

James A. Zimble, M.D.
President
Uniformed Services University of the
  Health Sciences

Other Invited Guests

Andrew Burness
Burness Communications

James F. Cawley, M.P.H.-P.A.-C
Associate Professor and
Director, PA/MPH Program
George Washington University
  Medical Center

Jack M. Colwill, M.D.
Professor and Chairman
Department of Family and Commu-
  nity Medicine
School of Medicine
University of Missouri-Columbia

Stephen E. Crane, Ph.D., M.P.H.
Deputy Director
Foundation for Health Services
  Research

Victoria del Corral
Manager, Programs and Conferences
Josiah Macy, Jr. Foundation

Henry Desmarais, M.D.
Principal
Health Policy Alternatives, Inc.

Joyce Emelio
Program Specialist
Bureau of Health Professions
U.S. Department of Health and
  Human Services

E. Harvey Estes, Jr., M.D.
Director
Reynolds Community Practitioner
  Program
North Carolina Medical Society
  Foundation

Gary Filerman, Ph.D.
Associate Director
Pew Health Professions Commission

Virginia Fowkes, M.H.S.
Program Director
PA Associates Program
Stanford University

Thomas Gaiter, M.D.
Medical Director
Howard University Hospital

Stephen Garfinkel
Writer/Editor

Nancy Gary, M.D.
Dean, F. Edward Hebert School of
  Medicine
The Uniformed Services University of
  the Health Sciences

Ruth Hanft, Ph.D.
Professor of Health Services
  Management and Policy
Department of Health Services
  Administration
George Washington University

Roderick Hooker, P.A., M.B.A.
Adjunct Investigator, Center for
  Health Services Research
Clinician, Department of Internal
  Medicine
Kaiser Permanente

Karen R. Matherlee
Co-Director
National Health Policy Forum

Thomas H. Meikle, Jr., M.D.
President
Josiah Macy, Jr. Foundation

Denis Oliver, Ph.D.
Professor and Director
Physician Assistant Program
University of Iowa

Sheila A. Ryan, Ph.D., R.N.
Dean of the School of Nursing and
Director, Medical Center Nursing
University of Rochester Medical
  Center

Edward S. Sekscenski, M.P.H.
Health Economist
Bureau of Health Professions
U.S. Department of Health and
  Human Services

Barbara Starfield, M.D., M.P.H.
Professor and Head, Division of
  Health Policy
School of Hygiene and Public Health
The Johns Hopkins University

AHC Staff

Roger J. Bulger, M.D.
President

Marian Osterweis, Ph.D.
Vice President

Elaine R. Rubin, Ph.D.
Program Associate

Stephen M. Merz
Research Assistant

Preface

HUMAN RESOURCE POLICY HAS BEEN A PRIORITY
area of the Association of Academic Health Centers (AHC) for some
time. Within the association, the Task Force on Human Resources for
Health has played a significant role in defining, studying, and evaluating a broad range of health workforce issues, including national
service for health professionals, nursing shortages, dental school
closures, interdisciplinary education, public health programs, and
allied health services.

Primary care has always emerged as a major concern in the task
force's studies and deliberations. Last year, for example, in its report,
Avoiding the Next Crisis in Health Care, the task force recommended
ways that academic health centers could play new roles to expand
access to health care services, to increase the numbers of primary care
providers, and to design innovative models for transforming the
primary care environment.

Knowing of the AHC's interest and expertise in human resource
issues, Dr. Thomas H. Meikle, Jr., president of the Josiah Macy, Jr.
Foundation, asked the association to conduct a workshop on the roles
of physician assistants and nurse practitioners in primary care. We are
grateful for the support and confidence of the foundation as the
workshop was a natural outgrowth of the task force's activities and
interest not only in primary care but also the national health care
reform agenda.

While health reform proposals are placing greater emphasis on
the delivery of primary care services, they do not appear to adequately
address human resource issues, particularly questions related to
nonphysician practitioners. The workshop furthers the public dialogue about primary care by focusing on those health professionals
currently viewed as physician substitutes in the primary care arena.

The workshop was designed to answer myriad questions about the
education, training, supply, demand, and practice patterns of physician assistants and nurse practitioners. While these practitioners have
been recognized as vital to the expansion of primary care services,
little appears to be known about their functions and the nature of

their educational and work environments. The questions are complex, and many issues require further research as workshop participants noted. However, the papers that follow provide a coherent, insightful review of these professions. We hope this book will help to expand the public debate on primary care and enhance the dialogue on human resource issues during this important era of change.

Again, let me thank the Josiah Macy, Jr. Foundation for its generous support as well as the many participants from across the health professions who contributed to the success of the workshop. Finally, I would like to thank Stephen Garfinkel for his fine editing of the manuscripts and Helen Schindler, AHC administrative assistant, for her excellent work in preparing the manuscript for publication.

D. Kay Clawson, M.D.
Executive Vice Chancellor
University of Kansas Medical Center
Chairman, AHC Task Force on Human Resources for Health

1

The Roles of Physician Assistants and Nurse Practitioners in Primary Care: An Overview of the Issues

Marian Osterweis and Stephen Garfinkel

THE ASSOCIATION OF ACADEMIC HEALTH CENTERS (AHC) convened a workshop to examine the educational, professional practice, and public policy issues that impact the ability of physician assistants and nurse practitioners to deliver primary care services and, if possible, to recommend actions to ensure that these practitioners are available to help to meet the nation's primary care needs, particularly in underserved areas.

The workshop brought together a group of approximately 35 health care leaders, policy experts, and analysts from academe, the private sector, and government. Physician assistants (PAs), nurse practitioners (NPs), and physicians representing the education and practice sectors were among the participants. Also participating were 15 chief executive officers of academic health centers, the institutions with major responsibilities for health professions education nationwide. These CEOs are also members of the AHC Task Force on Human Resources for Health, the AHC's expert group on human resource issues. This diverse group of participants represented a broad range of constituencies and perspectives on the myriad issues surrounding physician assistants, nurse practitioners, and primary care.

Participants were challenged to address the current and future roles for physician assistants and nurse practitioners in delivering primary care services, the educational and practice environments that shape these roles, and the public policies—from state practice laws to education to Medicare reimbursement—that require attention if greater numbers of people are to have access to primary care services.

The roles of physician assistants and nurse practitioners in primary care is a significant and timely topic, given the fast pace of the national health care reform agenda, the need to reevaluate primary care services and the contributions of nonphysicians in light of reform, and the potential for a dramatic increase in both the demand and utilization of these practitioners.

Several major, intertwined themes that emerged from the discussions were the interchangeability of roles and functions, primary care in underserved areas, educational reform, practice patterns, professional barriers, legal restraints, and consumer issues.

Roles and Functions

PAs and NPs have been providing health care in the United States for more than 25 years. Patients and doctors who have experience with these professionals speak highly of their skills. Evaluations of the care they provide are uniformly positive, suggesting that quality and outcomes are equivalent to those of physicians and in certain respects are superior. And, the literature indicates that these practitioners can substitute for physicians in as many as 75 to 90 percent of primary care functions.

Yet even people who are familiar with PAs and NPs have fundamental questions about them. Workshop participants raised such basic questions as, "What is the difference between what a PA can do and what an NP can do?" and "What can't PAs and NPs do that doctors can?"

Independence in practice is the most obvious feature that distinguishes physicians from nonphysician practitioners. Experts have noted that the most significant difference between PAs and NPs is not the skills they learn but the general orientation or socialization toward health care and the intensity of the desire for independent practice. Apparently, PAs are comfortable in a dependent role that requires physician supervision while nurses are striving to establish independent practice.

Physician assistants function in teams with physicians, most often playing supplementary or complementary roles. In fact, the legal basis of PA practice is physician dependence whereas NPs have resisted measures that would mandate physician supervision of their clinical practice activities. This difference, specifically the threat of independent NP practice in medical service delivery, has deeply colored perceptions about these practitioners. Nevertheless, in most clinical settings, NPs practice with some form of professional and legal connection to a physician practice, with legal and financial barriers precluding autonomous practice.

Other major determinants of roles are state practice laws and the delegatory styles and preferences of the employers and physicians with whom these practitioners work. When working in the same settings, however, PAs and NPs generally have the same job descriptions and perform the same roles. Hence, the confusion about the distinctions in PA and NP roles and competencies is well founded.

While both physician assistants and nurse practitioners have been known to substitute for physicians in providing primary care services, it appears that only a handful of studies has examined this role, particularly for nurses. Data provided by Roderick Hooker suggest considerable interchangeability of PAs and primary care physicians in an HMO but raise other issues about costs, referral patterns, and supervision needs.

It is clear, however, that nonphysicians make considerable contributions to primary health care, including follow-up on nonmedication therapies, counseling, patient management, and assessment of patient needs. Evaluations of the care PAs and NPs provide are uniformly positive, suggesting that quality and outcomes are equivalent to those of physicians and, in some respects, are superior. Workshop participants also pointed out that health care organizations can increase productivity and efficiency when these practitioners are utilized.

Training and Education

Nurse practitioners are licensed, registered nurses; the majority of PAs come from diverse backgrounds. Most PA programs were established by schools of medicine and offer a four-year baccalaureate degree (i.e., two years of general education and two years of clinical training). Educational preparation for NPs was established by schools of nursing, and the majority of programs are at the master degree level with NP students developing skills in advanced nursing practice.

Training programs for PAs and NPs offer certain advantages over physician training programs. Several participants pointed out that the cost of educating PAs and NPs is just a fraction of the cost of educating a physician, and that these practitioners take only two years to train.

In fact, Harvey Estes recommended streamlining and improving physician education by adopting some of the lessons learned from the PA training model. But he notes that implementing these reforms would likely take many years. In the meantime, as both Denis Oliver and Sheila Ryan point out, PA and NP training programs could substantially increase their output of graduates within a few years, given additional investment and other stimuli.

Currently one-third of the physician workforce (or 200,000 doctors) is in primary care, and there are 17,000 doctors graduating each year. By comparison, there are only 23,000 PAs in practice, of whom an estimated 60 percent are in primary care. The 55 PA programs graduated 1,600 PAs in 1992. An estimated 20,000–30,000 NPs with masters' degrees and certificates are in practice, and there are 3,500 graduates annually.

If we intend to train more PAs and NPs, a number of questions regarding their training programs must first be considered. The primary question is the overall aim of those programs. What should PAs be trained to do and what should NPs be trained to do? Should one or the other or both of these practitioners be trained to substitute for primary care physicians or should they be adjunct professionals? Should NPs be required to have a master's degree, as currently required by the American Nurses' Association, or is this requirement an example of degree inflation that results in more costly training of practitioners with no additional benefit to patients?

While no conclusive answers emerged on these issues, the questions stimulated broad debate. On one hand, participants recommended delineating the competencies that these practitioners are being trained to perform. On the other, participants, including Barbara Starfield, said competencies lead to a task-oriented approach rather than a role-oriented approach and thus preclude viewing PAs and NPs as potential substitutes for physicians.

Do we want both PAs and NPs to fill the same roles, and if so, what is the rationale for separate and distinct training programs? Some participants in the workshop favored the preservation of separate programs but recommended that all training include more multidisciplinary experiences with a variety of practitioners. There was debate, however, about how early in a program this team training should start and how much of total training should be in teams.

Participants proposed dramatic change with regard to training. Some participants proposed a fundamental reevaluation of the way we divide these primary care practitioners according to specialties or type of care. One suggestion was to organize training programs according to the type of care delivered, thus creating two distinct programs for PAs and NPs—one for primary care and one for specialty and acute care. Other participants proposed a training program for a generalist provider that would merge all primary care disciplines into a single program.

One of the problematic trends that may greatly affect primary care delivery is the use of PAs as substitutes for specialty medical residents in hospitals. James Cawley raised the issue, noting that this substitution diverts PAs from their intended roles in primary care, particularly in underserved areas. This trend is likely to become even more pronounced if President Clinton's health reform package includes the much-talked-about reduction in graduate medical education specialty slots.

Underserved Areas

Virginia Fowkes called attention to primary care delivery in underserved areas, emphasizing that the concerns about access to health care that spurred the development of the PA and NP professions 25 years ago are equally pressing today. Due to a variety of factors, including increased status, compensation, and provider reimbursement issues, PAs are duplicating the specialization and practice patterns of physicians. Among NPs, those educated in certificate programs are more likely to practice full time and to work in rural areas and small towns. Overall, NPs without a master's degree are more likely to be employed in primary health care and to practice in rural areas. Nevertheless, only a fraction of NPs are actually practicing in underserved areas.

State and federal reimbursement not only fails to correct the movement away from primary care in underserved areas but also contributes to it by providing differing rates of reimbursement to practitioners, whether PAs, NPs, or physicians, for the same services. In addition, the rates differ for the same services depending on whether the site of care is in an urban or rural setting.

Costs were also cited as a critical factor in the recruitment and retention of practitioners in underserved areas. Program survival often depends on state financial support. Participants noted that programs that placed graduates in underserved areas are often burdened with high operating costs to maintain sites over a wide geographic area. Expensive recruitment strategies due to location usually require outside financial support.

But the marketplace is not the only explanation. Restrictive scope-of-practice laws for nonphysician primary care providers also play a key role. These laws vary considerably from state to state, and states that allow PAs and NPs wider practice authority have a higher percentage of those practitioners in primary care.

Other workshop participants noted that changing demographics in the PA profession may also affect location. Formerly occupied mostly by males in mid-career, the PA profession now comprises younger women who are gravitating toward higher paying positions in urban areas.

Status, reward systems, and social and professional support are among the most significant determinants of recruitment to and retention in underserved areas. Participants noted the need to network services and sites to ensure successful and effective service delivery.

Finally, training may also play a significant role in attracting primary care practitioners to underserved areas. In the workshop as well as the papers, participants shared ideas about which training programs are most successful in this regard. Some participants questioned whether efforts to place graduates in underserved areas will only be overwhelmed by long-term retention problems. And overall, the question of which factors — reimbursement, scope-of-practice restrictions, demographics, or training — play the most influential roles remains unanswered.

Policy Questions

Given the potential for health reform to create a variety of sweeping changes, participants were encouraged to consider broad questions about how federal and state policies could be shaped to make the most efficient and effective use of non-physician primary care providers. Most important, how can policies be developed that take account of all health professions? How can policies be shaped to look beyond the generalist physician? How can institutional, professional, and governmental policies be altered to allow PAs and NPs to do what they have been trained to do? And how can public policies be used to encourage these practitioners to practice where they are most needed?

Certainly there is room for improvement. For example, current federal criteria for designating primary care health professional shortage areas do not account for the availability of nonphysician personnel. In the workshop and several of the papers, including that of Henry Desmarais, a wide variety of proposals was discussed to focus government policies more appropriately on these practitioners.

Numerous questions about the extent of federal government involvement and influence to determine scope of practice, quality, sites of care, allowable services, and reimbursement for PAs and NPs are at issue and unresolved. At the state level, scope of practice, including prescriptive authority, is the paramount issue.

Much discussion focused on the power of both the federal and state governments to influence the supply of and demand for these practitioners through reform policies that result in either managed care or single-payer systems. The following questions illustrate the major areas of concern:

- Should federal policies be developed to standardize state scope of practice laws, professional credentialing procedures, and reimbursement for PAs and NPs, or should policies vary from place to place?
- Should policies be drafted to boost incentives for PAs and NPs to practice primary care in underserved areas? If so, which incentives will be most effective?
- Should incentives be offered to schools and training sites to expand PA and NP training? If so, should these incentives focus on primary care only? Should they emphasize training for practice in underserved areas?
- Should government attempt to increase the number of PA and NP trainees by attempting to decrease the number of medical students? If so, should more PA training be done by medical schools that have the resources at hand or should programs in community colleges and other training sites continue to grow?
- Should all practitioners be paid equally for delivering the same services? If so, what is the most practical and cost-effective way to adjust current reimbursement rates? Would such adjustments raise overall health care costs and what might be other

possible unintended consequences of such a policy?

These questions are interrelated, and the order in which they are addressed could be extremely important. For example, it may be premature to determine how many PAs and NPs are needed to serve the nation's primary care needs before determining how best to attract these providers to the underserved areas where they are most needed.

Recommendations for Further Investigation

Conference participants were unable to agree about specific recommendations regarding the policies that should shape the training and utilization of physician assistants and nurse practitioners. The diversity of backgrounds and interests among the conferees added to the controversies over the appropriateness of change within the educational and provider environments. It was also difficult to make recommendations in areas that related to reimbursement and employers because these constituencies were not represented at the workshop.

Participants did agree, however, on the need for more information and recommended gathering more data on health care needs and the health care workforce. In addition, there was agreement on the need for innovation and change in education and practice to respond to a reformed health care environment.

Participants recommended in-depth research on a variety of issues, including national and local supply, workforce distribution, practice patterns, cost effectiveness, and accreditation and licensure. They identified a number of specific issues that need to be resolved before appropriate policy recommendations could be made, including:

- How many primary care providers are required to meet the nation's needs?
- How can practice laws be improved or changed to permit nonphysician practitioners to meet primary care needs?
- To what extent should physician assistants and nurse practitioners be used as physician substitutes, particularly in teaching hospitals?
- Should physician assistants and nurse practitioners perform the same roles and functions? What are the functions currently being performed by PAs and NPs in various settings?

- What is the ideal combination of primary care professionals working together in various settings, and what are the ideal roles for each of them to play?
- How well do PAs and NPs perform primary care functions compared to physicians, especially with regard to cost-effectiveness, clinical productivity, and patient care outcomes?

Participants acknowledged that health care reform is on a fast track with President Clinton's plan scheduled for release some time in fall 1993; policies will be developed, and perhaps implemented, before these questions are answered. Participants suggested that supply, scope of practice, practice, and reimbursement policies should be given top priority for the short term. Other issues where more research and analysis are required related to the educational environment, including quality measures for PA and NP programs, curricula, educational institutions, accreditation, and funding.

These questions will have to be answered in future research projects, conferences, and other association, professional, and institutional activities.

Conclusion

As the papers in this work demonstrate, an abundance of valuable literature has been produced to examine the roles and performance of PAs and NPs in primary care. But as these professions have matured, an abundance of new questions has emerged.

Health care reform will undoubtedly have a major impact on the urgency and complexity of the questions raised in these proceedings. Under our current health care system, PAs and NPs have proven that they can play a vital role in delivering primary care. It is up to us to continue to explore how we can maximize their effectiveness in a reformed health care environment.

2

Roles and Functions of Non-Physician Practitioners in Primary Care

Barbara Starfield

A NATIONALLY RESPECTED NURSE RESEARCHER HAS asserted that physicians have not risen to the challenges of primary care, even after 20 years of exhortation. Physicians, she averred, will never be interested in primary care. It's time for the responsibility to be given to nurses.[1]

A national survey of tasks carried out by physician assistants showed wide variability. In some areas, physician assistants were more likely to be functioning in specialty practice than in primary care. A major determinant of the nature of their role was not their training but whether the state in which they practice had prescriptive authority. States having prescriptive authority have a higher percentage of non-physician practitioners (NPPs) in primary care; those with no prescriptive authority are more likely to have NPPs in specialty care.[2] An article in the *American Journal of Public Health* documented how Mrs. B, a nurse working in her local community in western Massachusetts, could achieve all of the functions of primary care.[3]

Given such evidence of the suitability of non-physician providers for primary care practice, and given considerable sentiment toward their use in this manner, why has there been so little impetus for widespread movement towards such roles?

How Do Physician and Non-Physician Practitioner Roles Differ?

The most obvious difference between physicians and NPPs is the independence of their work. Physicians are individually licensed to practice medicine. Within that license, wide latitude is permitted in the nature and extent of their practice.

Much has been written about the extent of independence that should be accorded to NPPs; in general, they are assumed to be working under the supervision of, or at least in conjunction with, physicians. Within these constraints, there is little understanding of the nature of their contribution to the totality of health care.

One type of role is a substitute role, wherein NPPs take the place of physicians when there are no physicians available. An alternative is as a supplement to physicians, wherein physicians delegate functions to improve efficiency of care. A third alternative is a complementary role, wherein NPPs enhance the effectiveness of care by undertaking roles for which they are uniquely qualified.

When NPPs work in institutional or specialty settings, the purpose generally is a supplementary one; they carry out roles that are part of the overall function of the physicians with whom they work. However, the nature and variability of their role in primary care is unclear.

The lack of understanding of the role of non-physician personnel in primary care practice is hardly surprising, given the similar lack of understanding of primary care practice by physicians. Few can specify how primary care practice differs from the practice of specialists, and there may indeed be a considerable amount of overlap, to the great detriment of quality, accessibility, and costs of care.

A Review of the Literature

Most of the literature on physician assistants and nurse practitioners dates back to the 1970s,[4] a period when physician supply was believed to be inadequate and when there appeared to be lessons from the experiences of approaches such as the "barefoot doctors." Unfortunately, this literature lacks the conceptual underpinnings that are required for an analysis of policy options for the primary care practice of NPPs.

The existing literature gives little guidance on the extent to which non-physician practitioners provide primary care. A bibliography compiled in 1991 and entitled "Nursing in Primary Care" included about 120 articles with primary care stated or implied in their titles, culled from more than 400 papers in 60 journals from 1987 to 1990.[5] The chosen articles represented demonstration projects, intervention studies, educational programs, and the views of nursing leaders. The vast majority dealt with developing countries. About a dozen were limited to midwifery. Only three dealt with nurses as independent providers. The remainder dealt with nurses as members of a team. That is, only a handful of studies examined nurses in a substitute role; the great majority dealt with nurses in a supplementary or complementary role.

A very recent meta-analysis of publications dealing with primary care nursing roles identified 38 articles that involved nurse practitioners in an intervention in the United States or Canada; a control group involving physician-only care; a measure of effect in terms of processes of care, clinical outcomes or utilization/cost-effectiveness; and data that permitted calculation of effect size.[6] The conclusions follow.

Nurses were found to provide more health promotion activities, score higher on quality-of-care measures, order a greater number of — but less expensive — laboratory tests, and have equivalent rates of drug prescribing. They achieved higher scores on resolution of patients' problems and better functional status of patients, scored better on measures of patient satisfaction and patient compliance, and had equivalent scores to physicians on patient knowledge. Nurses spent 50 percent more time with patients and had an equivalent number of visits per patient. Their patients experienced fewer hospitalizations, and the average cost per visit was lower (when cost included salaries of the individual providing care).

The findings were confirmed by a sub-analysis of studies in which patients were randomly assigned, thus controlling for possible effect of case-mix differences between the patients of physicians and those of nurses. The meta-analysis concluded that nurses practicing in "advanced practice roles" are cost-effective providers of primary care services.

Thus, when primary care is viewed as a collection of services consisting of specific aspects of diagnosis and management *not necessarily unique to primary care*, there is at least some evidence that non-physicians can make a considerable contribution. If the functions are also characteristic of specialty care, then the evidence might equally well support the role of NPPs in specialty care.

Furthermore, some important characteristics of the process of primary care were not included in any of these studies. Among these are rates of referral, which are a key factor when considering the role of a primary care practitioner. The critical question is whether NPPs can carry out the functions of *primary care*. In order to answer this question, it is necessary to consider the functions and tasks of primary care.

Functions in Primary Care

Primary care is that level of services that bears responsibility for the vast majority — perhaps 99 percent — of the health problems of the population in any given area. In order to fulfill that responsibility, primary care has four unique functions: it is first-contact care, it is longitudinal over time, it is comprehensive, and it is the coordinator of care.[7]

First contact means that care has to be provided when it is needed. Services must be accessible in time and place, and by financing and culture. This accessibility must be manifested as a behavior; the population must use the source of care in a timely manner when a need for care is perceived.

Longitudinal means that care is time-oriented rather than oriented to a disease or a disease episode. Longitudinal care is focused on a person rather than on a problem or type of problem. There must be at least an informal agreement of the patient to enroll as a regular patient and of the practitioner to be the regular source of care. Moreover, it must be demonstrated that care is sought from the same source each time it is needed, except for specific referrals made by the primary care source to other types of providers.

Comprehensive means that there is an assumed responsibility to provide care for the most common 99 percent of problems in the population. An explicit and appropriately inclusive range of services must be available, and the services must be provided when they are needed.

Coordination is the function that puts the pieces together when patients are sent elsewhere for referrals, procedures, or therapies. The coordinating function requires some mechanism of continuity to provide the information about the care patients receive elsewhere, and it also requires recognition of information generated when patients must be seen elsewhere for various aspects of their care.

What Are the Tasks Related to These Functions?

Figure 1 specifies the components of the health services system in terms that can be translated into tasks. In this conceptualization, the structure is that aspect of the system that provides the potential for activities. These activities, or processes, are an interaction between practitioners and patients, or between facilities and populations.

Activities contributed by practitioners or facilities include the recognition of needs (including those for preventive services, symp-

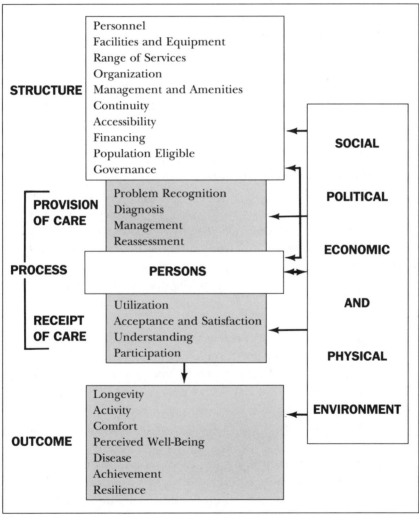

Figure 1
The Health Services System

toms, ongoing health problems or dispositions resulting from visits elsewhere), the process of diagnosis, management (including hospitalizations, medications, counseling and other non-medication therapies) and the process of reassessment (which involves feedback concerning the earlier steps). On the patient's (or population's) side, the activities include use of services, acceptance, satisfaction with services, understanding of ministrations, and participation in care — from the more passive participation, known as compliance, to active involvement in changing therapy when doing so seems appropriate.

The third component of the health system concerns the outcomes of care. These outcomes are influenced by the processes of the health system in interaction with the impact of all aspects of the environment on health status.

This conceptualization pertains to all levels of the health system, not only primary care. However, it can be used to characterize each of the four components of services that are uniquely primary care. Doing so requires the specification of one structural element to provide the potential for an activity and one process element to convert the potential into a behavior.

First contact, for example, requires that the facility or practitioner be accessible; it also requires that the patient (or population) actually use those particular services (rather than going elsewhere) each time a new need is perceived. Longitudinality requires that the facility or practitioner define the eligible population (the structural element). It also requires that the individuals in the population actually use the services over time for non-referred care, regardless of the type of problem.

Comprehensiveness requires, as the potential, that the services or practitioner define the range of services that are to be provided and that this range be broad enough to encompass the most common needs experienced by that particular population. The other problems will require referral, as they will occur too infrequently in the population of a primary care practice for the practitioner to maintain competence.

Coordination, the fourth primary care component, is represented by the structural element of continuity; this continuity (which is generally achievable by some combination of individuals, teams, medical record, computers, or client-held records) is necessary for information about patients or populations to be transferred from one

16

place to another. The behavioral element of coordination is the recognition of this information by the ongoing practitioner or primary care team. This recognition is necessary for a primary care facility to "put it all together" for the patient.

These four combinations of structural and process elements constitute primary care; they would *not* be expected in secondary or tertiary care.

How Well Can NPPs Perform These Functions?

Non-physician practitioners might carry out any of the many functions, or multiple functions, within this model of the elements of care. *However, to enhance primary care uniquely, they must contribute to one or more of the four elements enumerated above.*

There is evidence that NPPs perform somewhat better than physicians in recognizing certain kinds of problems experienced by patients. These include, for example, follow-up on non-medication therapies that have previously been prescribed for patients. In general, they appear to be superior to physicians in managing patients whose care requires counseling, although physicians appear to be superior in managing care requiring technical solutions.[8]

There is also some evidence that non-physician practitioners provide services in geographic areas that otherwise lack such services. Physician assistants, in particular, are more willing to locate in non-affluent, medically underserved areas with higher percentages of non-white individuals.[9] The literature on acceptance of, and satisfaction with, care provided by non-physician professionals is mixed, but most studies have not been conducted with the patients blinded to the training of the practitioner under study.

In general, it may be inferred (though it has not been demonstrated) that some aspects of primary care might be better achieved by non-physician practitioners than by physicians.

First-contact care may be achieved at a higher level by non-physician practitioners if their increased availability is translated into a heightened willingness of people to consult them directly rather than to go to alternative sources of care, such as emergency rooms.

Longitudinality of care might be enhanced if non-physician practitioners are more person-focused, and if people are more willing to engage them, rather than physicians, in dealing with the wide variety of problems experienced over time.

The evidence regarding comprehensiveness is sparse; whether or not non-physician practitioners are well enough trained to offer services for and deal with the wide range of problems presenting in primary care is unknown. What evidence there is suggests that NPPs may function better in complementary roles to physicians rather than as substitutes in this component of primary care. That is, they may be better than physicians in providing certain types of services, especially those relating to recognition of the need for and provision of non-technical services.

As coordinators of care, non-physician practitioners may be superior to physicians and thus complement the physician's role. They appear to be better in recognizing certain types of information about patients than are physicians. However, the one study that examined recognition of information about patients from visits that patients made elsewhere is not encouraging in this regard. Nurse practitioners functioned equally poorly to physicians in that they recognized only a minority of visits that patients made elsewhere in the interval between two scheduled visits.[10]

Thus, the evidence seems to suggest an NPP role that is supplementary and complementary to that of physicians. Whether NPPs do as well as, or better than, physicians in a substitute primary care role is not clear.

Deployment of NPPs in Primary Care

In the mid 1980s, there were 18.5 NPPs per 100,000 population; in rural areas there were 15 per 100,000. In three large HMOs, the rate was 27 per 100,000, but there was marked variability in their deployment across the HMOs. In adult primary care, this variability ranged from involvement in 6 percent of visits to 47 percent; in general pediatrics, NPPs were involved in no visits in one HMO, 7 percent in another, and 26 percent in the third. HMOs that involved NPPs in a relatively high proportion of visits did so consistently across the two primary care specialties, as well as obstetrics and gynecology. Only one HMO involved NPPs in specialty care visits and did so to a very high degree (45 percent to 60 percent of visits, depending on specialty). This was the same HMO that made greatest use of NPPs in primary care.[11]

An important issue is the extent to which NPPs can be expected to undertake the totality of primary care, achieving all of its four functions. NPPs may function as formal primary care givers in developing countries where health service needs differ substantially from those in industrialized countries. In many industrialized countries, NPPs have formal roles in primary care, functioning as part of a team, usually in roles complementary to physicians. For example, nurses provide much of the outreach services in well-child supervision in Scandinavia and the Netherlands.[12]

The United States appears to be a fine setting for studies of the usefulness of NPPs as substitute primary care providers. Many managed care organizations have restrictions on the extent to which enrolled patients may see physicians; patients often have to provide special justification for an appointment with a physician rather than an NPP. However, little is known about the extent to which these managed care organizations achieve the elements of primary care and the extent to which the NPPs that they employ contribute to achieving those elements.

In the face of rapidly declining interest in primary care practice among physicians in the United States, many advocates for NPPs assert that primary care should be a nursing specialty rather than a physician specialty. If this is the case, and if the argument is extended to other NPPs, these new roles will have to address the four unique and essential features of primary care. An appropriate first step appears to be evaluating current functions of NPPs, including the extent to which they bear responsibility for each of the four features and for the four in combination. Once accomplished, these studies could provide direction to a reassessment of future education and deployment of NPPs, either as supplements or complements to physicians in primary care or, alternatively, as substitutes for physicians who, as a group, are abdicating this role within the health services system.

References

1. Starfield B. *Primary Care: Concept Evaluation and Policy.* New York, NY: Oxford University Press; 1992.
2. Willis J. Barriers to physician assistant practice in primary care and medically underserved areas: background. Presented at the Third Annual Primary Care Conference, Agency for Health Care Policy and Research; January 11-12, 1993; Atlanta, Ga.
3. Dreher M. District nursing: the cost benefits of a population-based practice. *Am J Public Health.* 1984;74:1107-11.
4. Brown S, Grimes D. A meta-analysis of process of care, clinical outcomes, and cost-effectiveness of nurses in primary care roles: nurse practitioners and nurse-midwives. Presented at the Third Annual Primary Care Conference, Agency for Health Care Policy and Research; January 11-12, 1993; Atlanta, Ga.

5. D'Angelo L. Bibliography on nursing in primary care. (Manuscript) University of Pennsylvania; 1991.

6. Brown S, Grimes D. A meta-analysis of process of care, clinical outcomes, and cost-effectiveness of nurses in primary care roles: nurse practitioners and nurse-midwives. Presented at the Third Annual Primary Care Conference, Agency for Health Care Policy and Research; January 11-12, 1993; Atlanta, Ga.

7. Starfield B. *Primary Care: Concept Evaluation and Policy.* New York, NY: Oxford University Press; 1992.

8. United States Congress, Office of Technology Assessment. *Nurse Practitioners, Physician Assistants, and Certified Nurse-Midwives: A Policy Analysis.* Washington, DC: U.S. Government Printing Office; 1986. Case Study 37.

9. United States Congress, Office of Technology Assessment. *Nurse Practitioners, Physician Assistants, and Certified Nurse-Midwives: A Policy Analysis.* Washington, DC: U.S. Government Printing Office; 1986. Case Study 37.

10. Simborg D, Starfield B, Horn S. Physician and non-physician health practitioners: the characteristics of their practice and their relationships. *Am J Public Health.* 1978;68:44-48.

11. Weiner J, Steinwachs D, Williamson J. Nurse practitioner and physician assistant practices in three HMOs: implications for future U.S. health manpower needs. *Am J Public Health.* 1986;76:507-11.

12. Starfield B, Harlow J. Cross-national comparisons of well-child supervision. (Manuscript) The Johns Hopkins University; 1993.

3

Physician Assistants in the Health Care Workforce

James F. Cawley

As THE NATION DEBATES VARIOUS HEALTH CARE RE-
form proposals, attention has focused on issues related to America's
health workforce. Concern for the looming cost implications of the
generalist/specialist imbalance and the limits on health care access
resulting from uneven provider distribution — problems that have
existed since the 1960s — has spurred renewed interest in issues such
as the future supply of primary care providers.

Proposed reforms seek to improve the accessibility, efficiency,
and availability of primary care and tend to focus on changing the
size, structure, and financing of graduate medical education (GME).
Approaches include increasing incentives for medical school graduates to select generalist careers, expanding medical student loan
forgiveness and national service programs, increasing amounts of
primary care training experiences for physician residents, shifting
Medicare GME funds away from overcrowded specialty programs, and redirecting these funds to generalist and primary care
education.[1]

A complementary approach also receiving attention in policy
circles is expanding utilization of non-physician health providers.
Physician assistants (PAs), along with nurse practitioners (NPs) and
certified nurse-midwives, perform medical diagnostic and therapeutic functions at lower costs than physicians. They are trained to
provide primary care services, but they are capable of assuming
specialty roles. And they improve health care quality, productivity,
and access.[2]

PAs and NPs are considered essential partners, along with family physicians, general internists, and general pediatricians, in America's primary care workforce.[3] Research suggests that health care organizations employing a proper mix of physician and non-physician providers may be more effective in delivering primary care and achieving cost savings than those employing older forms of practice arrangements.[4] Yet until recently, there has been little discussion of health workforce strategies incorporating the potential of PAs to improve efficiency and reduce cost. Many aspects of PAs' current clinical practice activities have not been addressed, and the number of PAs that would be needed to meet future health professions workforce requirements has not been calculated.

Practice Economics

PAs in primary care have proven capable of managing about three-fourths of the clinical problems encountered in ambulatory settings. Some economists have termed this figure the MD/PA substitutability ratio. They have pointed out that this ratio may vary according to practice specialty or practice setting.

PA productivity seems optimal in ambulatory practices and organized settings, such as health maintenance organizations, where PA performance has been carefully measured.[5] Record's work and data from other studies suggest that the most influential factors on PA clinical productivity are the task delegation and supervision behaviors of employing physicians.[6]

This finding was also observed in a recent examination of non-physician staffing and utilization in the Veterans Administration (VA) hospital system. The Institute of Medicine conducted a study in 1992 that addressed future medical staffing requirements for the VA system (172 hospitals, 68 satellite outpatient clinics, 127 nursing homes) and contained data describing staffing policies and utilization patterns of four types of non-physicians: PAs, NPs, clinical nurse specialists, and nurse anesthetists. The study observed the clinical activities of these professionals in multiple settings and measured their opinions regarding professional duties with a standardized questionnaire.

The study indicated that non-physicians appeared to be underutilized in the VA system. It recommended that physicians receive better orientation regarding non-physician capabilities and roles, and that they develop appropriate clinical delegation skills.

This recommendation derived from the study's finding that supervising physicians' attitudes and styles of task delegation tended to determine the most effective utilization patterns of non-physicians — more than the education and clinical skill levels of these providers.[7]

Legal concerns and provider reimbursement issues can also affect PA utilization and effectiveness in primary care practices. Uneven state medical practice acts, the lack of authorization to prescribe medications, and the absence of Medicare and private third-party reimbursement in many ambulatory settings (exceptions being health professions shortage areas, medically underserved areas, and Medicare-approved rural health clinics) restrict PA utilization. Altering these practice barriers would improve PA capabilities to extend care, particularly in primary care.

Data on PA productivity and physician substitutability in inpatient settings and accurate information describing PA activities and potentials in GME programs are generally lacking, yet several proven staffing models exist. Large teaching hospitals, typically located in Eastern states, employ sizable numbers of PAs as part of their inpatient medical house staff. Montefiore Hospital in the Bronx has used PAs for more than 20 years and employs more than 150, most of them in roles that previously belonged to residents. Montefiore sponsors innovative "PA residency" programs in surgery and obstetrics/gynecology and has balanced its physician residency program output in these and other specialties by employing a mix of PAs and physician residents.

These clinical educational opportunities have emerged from experiences using PAs in GME programs that meld hospital clinical service needs with advanced training opportunities for PAs in specialties; they also provide institutions with a supply of well-trained medical personnel.[8] Using PAs in these roles improves continuity of care, enriches educational experiences for residents and reduces overall costs.[9]

Examples of effective use of PAs in GME substitution roles exist in similar urban-based teaching hospitals, academic health centers, medium-sized community hospitals that have phased out residency programs, and other tertiary care institutions. For example, Geisinger Medical Center, a 536-bed referral facility in rural northeastern Pennsylvania, employs more than 110 PAs, many in GME-related roles, in which they have demonstrated clinical versatility and multi-specialty expertise.[10]

Several recent papers have described the safety, quality of clinical care, cost effectiveness and, in some cases, improved clinical outcomes when PAs are used on hospital teaching services. While it has been mistakenly stated that PA capabilities in inpatient settings extend only to non-critical care areas,[11] a number of studies have clearly demonstrated PA safety and clinical efficacy when utilized in a wide range of inpatient clinical roles, including inpatient medical and surgical units,[12] emergency departments,[13] angiography suites,[14] critical care units,[15] subspecialty services,[16] and endoscopy units.[17]

No one has directly measured PA clinical productivity rates and PAs' capacity to substitute for physicians in inpatient roles. In health maintenance organizations, PAs have been shown to be capable of delivering roughly 63 percent of the medical care services required at no loss of quality of care and at 38 percent of the cost of physicians.[18]

Recently, Hooker reported data that compared clinical productivity rates of both PAs and NPs with those of primary care physicians, using outpatient visits as the unit of measure. In internal medicine, PAs saw a mean of 19.0 patients per day — more than MDs (17.4) or NPs (17.0). In family practice, rates were 22.5 per day for MDs and 21.5 for both PAs and NPs; in pediatrics, rates were 22.3 for PAs, 18.7 for NPs, and 16.25 for MDs.[19] These data further confirm that PA and NP clinical productivity, as demonstrated in ambulatory practices in organized settings with team approaches and structured division of staffing, compares favorably to that of physicians. While it seems probable that similar rates of clinical efficiency (physician substitutability) should exist when PAs are used in inpatient settings, more studies should be done examining PA performance in such roles.

Economic analysis of the utilization of advanced practice nurses in hospital settings indicates that these and perhaps other types of non-physicians are underutilized in health services delivery;[20] projections of potential cost savings by increasing use of non-physicians are considerable.[21]

Practice Specialty and Setting

After a decade in which PAs were largely deployed in primary care, more recent utilization patterns reveal a steady trend toward practice in non-primary care specialties and urban settings. While PAs are still more likely to practice in primary care and medically underserved areas than are physicians, the number of PAs working in primary care specialties has fallen steadily over the past 15 years. Among practicing PAs, only 43 percent currently work in family practice, general internal medicine, and general pediatrics – down from 57 percent in 1980 (see Table 1). Only 32 percent are in family practice.[23]

As the proportion of PAs in primary care declined, the rates of PAs working in acute care settings, specialties, and subspecialties rose correspondingly. Even as the PA profession was rapidly expanding in size, the percentage of PAs employed in hospital settings increased from 14 percent in 1980 to nearly 30 percent in 1993.

For many hospitals, residency program cutbacks, curtailed availability of international medical graduates (IMGs), and cost considerations were key factors leading to expanded inpatient roles for PAs. Often, PAs were used where they essentially substituted for physician residents.[24] Currently, about 28 percent of all PAs, or approximately 6,500, are employed in full-time inpatient care settings. In a sample of 1,690 hospital PAs recently surveyed, 45 percent identify themselves as "house officers." Other hospital PAs work in specialty or outpatient clinics or in departments such as employee health or emergency services. More than 90 percent have medical staff privileges, written job descriptions, and permission to write diagnostic and therapeutic orders. PA inpatient practice tends to be focused in specialty care, with 19.4 percent in surgical subspecialties, 18.6 per-

---

Table 1

Specialty Distribution of PAs by Percentage, 1974-1992.

	1974	1978	1981	1984	1987	1992
Specialty	N =939	3,416	4,312	6,552	10,692	13,500
Family Practice*	43.6	52.0	49.1	42.5	38.7	131.4
General Internal Medicine*	20.0	12.0	8.9	9.2	9.5	8.9
General Pediatrics*	6.2	3.3	3.4	4.1	4.0	2.5
General Surgery	12.1	5.5	4.6	5.1	8.8	8.0
Surgical Subspecialties	6.8	6.2	7.7	12.5	13.8	21.7
Emergency Medicine	1.3	4.9	4.5	6.4	6.5	8.0
Medical Subspecialties	3.9	6.3	2.7	4.8	7.1	9.4
Occupational Medicine	1.8	2.7	3.1	4.1	4.1	3.9
Other	4.3	7.1	16.0	11.3	7.5	6.9

*Primary care specialties

Sources: Association of Physician Assistant Programs, American Academy of Physician Assistants, and Health Resources and Services Administration, U.S. Department of Health and Human Services.

Table 2

Trends in DA Practice Setting (Percentages), 1981-1992.

	1981	1984	1987	1992
N=	4,312	6,552	3,309	13,173
Private Office[1]	35.8	34.5	33.2	32.7
Hospital	29.5	31.3	28.6	30.9
Ambulatory Clinic[2]	24.9	17.7	17.0	17.8
Health Maintenance Organization	N/A	N/A	6.9	7.2
Military	9.4	7.3	7.6	6.0
Other	0.4	9.2	6.7	12.6

Sources: Association of Physician Assistant Programs and American Academy of Physician Assistants.

[1] Either solo or group practice
[2] Includes community-based public, privately-sponsored, inner city, substance abuse, student health, correctional medicine, and rural health clinics.

cent in medical subspecialties, 14.8 percent in emergency medicine, and 9.5 percent in general surgery.[25]

Distribution patterns of PAs by practice setting have been stable, with roughly one-third working in group practices and health maintenance organizations, a bit fewer in hospitals, and the remainder in clinics, solo private practices, and military or other institutional settings (see Table 2).[26]

While PA distribution spans the gamut of medical specialties and practice settings, there are notable geographic differences in practice patterns. Overall, PA state-by-state distribution roughly parallels that of the population, but PA practice in Western states tends more often to be in office-based, ambulatory, and primary care practices, whereas in Eastern states, it is far more common for PAs to practice in acute care hospitals, inpatient specialties, and other institutionally based settings.

In one cohort of over 11,000 PAs, the percentage in primary care practices in Western states was 77 percent, versus 48 percent in Eastern states; only 13.9 percent of PAs in Western states were working in hospital and institutional settings, versus 45.5 percent in Eastern states.[27] Surveys of PAs practicing in some Eastern states, such as New York, Pennsylvania, and Maryland, indicate that more than half of all PAs in these states work in inpatient hospital roles. These practice differences stem from the multiple, sometimes competing, medical marketplace demands that emerged for PAs in different regions, as well as federally sponsored PA educational and deployment strategies.

In 1981, 27 percent of PAs were in practice in communities of less than 10,000 population; in 1992, the percentage was 16 percent. Since nearly all rural PAs are in primary care (86.6 percent), factors influencing the trend away from primary care and rural practice often overlap. These include the retirement of older male PAs (who were more likely than women to enter practices in underserved areas), the increasing proportion of women in the profession (43 percent of the practicing PA population in 1992; 60 percent of currently enrolled students), and the strong demand and higher remuneration in specialty and hospital practices.[28]

In many ways, PA utilization patterns over the last decade have closely mirrored those of physicians. As the physician workforce became increasingly specialized, evolving patterns of physician behaviors and changes in the division of medical labor have influenced PA utilization in the same direction. Demand for PAs remains strong across the board, and salaries have risen accordingly over the past five to seven years; the mean salary level for PAs in 1992 for all practice specialties was approximately $48,000 (higher in specialty areas and lower in primary care).[29] For the future, incentives should be considered that would allow primary care practices to better compete with hospital, institutional, and specialty employers in seeking PA services.

Expanding PA Supply

Interest in increasing the utilization of PAs and other non-physicians as providers of primary care in medically underserved areas and populations has returned to pre-GMENAC (Graduate Medical Education National Advisory Committee) levels.[22] Increasing the supply of PAs seems to be a rational way to ensure a steady supply of PAs for roles in augmenting primary care. It remains a federal health policy priority to educate and use PAs in primary care roles where they have proven to be safe and capable providers. Since physicians continue to avoid primary care fields, PAs represent an effective means of improving access in underserved areas. Future health professions planning should insure that an adequate number of PAs is supplied for employment in primary care practice settings.

The nation's 55 accredited PA educational programs graduated

1,600 students in 1992, up by several hundred from 1991. The typical PA program is a two-year curriculum awarding the bachelor's degree, is set in an academic health center or university, employs five to six full-time faculty, has an annual budget of approximately $470,000, and enrolls an average of 30 students per class.

In 1992, the Division of Medicine in the Health Resources and Services Administration's Bureau of Health Professions awarded a total of $5 million to 34 programs under the Title VII PA Grants Program for Physician Assistants. The grant program's priorities focus on primary care education and offer incentives for programs whose graduates enter primary care practice or locate in medically underserved areas. Recently, more than half of all PA program graduates selected employment positions in primary care, after several years in which the rate of primary care selection dipped.[30]

It has been suggested that the supply of PAs may need to be doubled or even tripled in the coming years to meet anticipated demand in primary care roles.[31] Current authorization levels for Title VII PA Grant Program funding would permit $7.5 million to be available in 1994 and $9 million in 1995. These increases should allow for the expansion of enrollment in existing PA programs and provide start-up funds for academic health centers or universities seeking to sponsor PA programs. They would enable educational programs in various stages of development (about a dozen, most of which are not set in academic health centers) to become fully functional. They would also support activities required by expansion of PA education, such as faculty development and recruitment efforts and the broadening of the clinical training affiliations of PA educational programs. Under current law, authority is granted to increase Title VII funding of PA education over the next several years, and based upon conservative estimates of educational program output, the annual supply of PA graduates could be raised to 3,500 by the year 2000 — bringing the total number of PAs in clinical practice to 42,700 (see Table 3).

PAs and GME Reform

As policy makers consider reforms that would change methods of GME financing and structure, PAs may play an increasingly important role in augmenting medical care services in hospital-based settings. PA utilization in hospital-based roles, particularly in institutions sponsoring GME programs, has become common. PAs, to a greater

Table 3
Projected Supply of Physician Assistants, 1993-2000.

Year	PA Education Graduates*	Total Practicing PAs**
1993	1,800	24,800
1994	1,800	26,600
1995	2,000	28,000
1996	2,300	30,300
1997	2,600	32,900
1998	3,000	35,900
1999	3,300	39,200
2000	3,500	42,700

*Based on the appropriation of maximally authorized levels of PA Grant Program support under Section 750 of Title VII from 1993 to 1995 and continuation of this level through 2000, allowing the expansion of existing programs and the development of 10 to 20 additional programs.

**Estimates assume 1 percent attrition.

degree than NPs, are employed in teaching hospitals essentially to substitute for physician residents. Employing PAs allows these institutions and academic health centers to adjust resident numbers without affecting clinical service coverage. This approach balances resident numbers in GME programs and compensates for hospital clinical service loss of residents. While PAs are trained for roles in primary care, they have readily adapted to inpatient roles, showing clinical competency in maintaining quality patient care.[32]

If the goal of achieving a 50-50 balance of specialist-generalist physician distribution in the United States is to be achieved soon, changing the GME system to produce more generalist physicians will be necessary. By shifting monies within Medicare's $5.2 billion subsidy to graduate medical education, policy makers hope to slow the proliferation of subspecialization, promote the selection of generalist careers by medical school graduates, and raise the status of primary care in medical education and practice.[33]

It has been suggested that residency slots in the future be limited to 115 percent of the number of annual allopathic medical graduates. This limit would eliminate about 11,000 slots from the roughly 80,000 existing residency positions. Less support would go to residency programs in certain specialties and subspecialties; more would go toward primary care education. Transferred funds could also be used for expansion of loan and loan-for-service plans for medical and health professions students under the National Health Service Corps.

In 1991, another development occurred which will likely herald changes in graduate medical education and accelerate the already strong demand for PAs in hospital settings. As state regulatory agencies, following New York's lead, impose limitations on the maximum number of work hours of physician residents, hospitals will have to maintain existing levels of clinical care with less resident availability.

Thorpe examined the impact of these limitations on teaching hospitals and estimated the costs of compensating for losses in resident coverage. Enlisting attending physicians to replace residents (which would cost $160 million) or hiring licensed physicians as house officers would be expensive options. He estimated that a mix of PAs and physician residents could provide the necessary coverage of inpatient services for far less ($85 million). While the option of using PAs would be less costly than other staffing alternatives, it would require about 1,300 additional PAs for New York teaching hospitals alone, and hospitals already have difficulty attracting enough PAs.[34]

In internal medicine, residency programs are preparing to "downsize" in response to several interacting forces: the prediction of an oversupply of physicians, a service-driven GME system, the growth of specialization, and the diminishing attraction of this specialty for recent medical graduates. As internal medicine programs reduce their size, teaching hospitals will adjust staffing of inpatient teaching services using a combination of physician residents, international medical graduates, and PAs.[35]

Findings relevant to this issue have begun to appear, although good measures of the specific capacities of PAs and other non-physicians in roles replacing physician residents have yet to be precisely determined. In a time motion study involving two non-physicians and eight internal medicine residents in two New York City teaching hospitals, Knickman, Lipkin, and colleagues observed the medical tasks traditionally performed by physician residents and projected several inpatient staffing models to determine their potential for resident substitution. They classified inpatient clinical activities into three categories: those that had to be done by physicians, those that were educational only, and those that could be done by non-physicians. The researchers recorded a total of 1,726 activities.

Under a model in which the physician is the primary medical manager of the patient, residents spend about half of their time on activities that must be done by a physician. Under an alternative model, in which the non-physician — in this instance an NP — would assume responsibility for the day-to-day monitoring of the patient, only 20 percent of activities would require a physician. The study concluded that there is substantial potential for non-physicians to assume inpatient medical tasks and that only 20 percent of each resident's lost time needs to be replaced with other physicians' time. To achieve this level of efficiency, hospitals would need to restructure their inpatient staffing models.[36]

The trend of using PAs as resident substitutes raises several issues. There is a relatively small number of PAs produced at present, and expanding PA utilization in GME roles diverts them from intended roles in primary care and medically underserved settings. The current U.S. Department of Health and Human Services mandate for the educational orientation and practice utilization of these health professionals strongly emphasizes a primary care focus and intends that PA health personnel contributions be directed to extend primary care services and improve health access.

A second issue involves the clinical service needs of teaching hospitals that are or will be cutting their numbers of physician residents. These institutions are concerned about ways to receive Medicare reimbursement for PA employment costs in the face of less GME resident subsidy payments. Teaching hospitals sponsoring GME programs are now compensated for their medical education activities under Medicare direct and indirect payments. If residency positions are cut, hospitals face the loss of both Medicare revenue and clinical staffing. Hospitals that have employed PAs to augment physician and resident services in GME programs have compensated for the loss of Medicare GME funding by incorporating the following into their budgets:

- The reimbursable revenue generated by PAs in providing general inpatient clinical services, which include laboratory tests and clinical procedures. Estimates of revenue generation potential for these tests and procedures range from two- to three-fold higher than employment costs.
- Reimbursement obtained for PA clinical services under Medicare Part B. The law allows for reimbursement for PA services at 65 percent of physician rates for assisting at surgery, 75 percent for services performed in a hospital, and 85 percent for

those performed in a nursing home. Prior to approval of PA eligibility under Medicare Part B, established in 1986 (P.L. 99-509), hospitals usually recovered PA employment costs within per diem charges billed under Medicare DRG-based Part A allowances. It is believed that some hospitals continue to finance their use of PAs through this mechanism.

Another consideration is that neither PA educational programs nor teaching hospitals have many financial incentives to participate in the clinical education of PA students. With PA grant program funding targeted specifically toward primary care, it would be difficult for most existing programs to rapidly expand production of PAs for inpatient roles. If PAs are expected to fulfill resident substitute positions, it may be necessary to secure the assistance of teaching centers either to develop more clinical training experiences for PA students or to sponsor PA programs. Educational support for PAs could require that mechanisms linking Medicare GME training funds be used to compensate teaching institutions that shift the direction of medical educational from specialty areas toward primary care.

Changing Roles: PAs, NPs, and MDs

In many research studies and health professions planning discussions, PAs and NPs are regarded as virtually interchangeable in their clinical roles and practice capabilities. While they appear to be equivalent providers in their scope of practice, and indeed in many clinical settings they are, PAs and NPs possess distinctly different educational and professional orientations. These differences have cast them in diverging roles in clinical practice and hold implications for their future.

The major difference between NPs and PAs is their stance on scope-of-practice limits and their legal and professional relationships with physicians. NPs resist measures that would mandate physician supervision of their clinical practice, stating that they are separately licensed health professionals who do not require physician involvement in their practice. In contrast, the legal basis of PA practice is physician dependence.

Consequently, physicians perceive a potential threat in independent NP practice and firmly oppose the idea through the American Medical Association and other physician groups. In most clinical settings, NP practice exists within some form of professional and legal connection to physician practice, and various legal and financial barriers usually preclude the economic viability of autonomous NP practice. In managed care settings and organized government systems, role differences between PAs and NPs do not pose problems, since both groups are used in structured roles, and physicians and non-physicians work as salaried employees. In private practice settings, sensitivities between NPs and MDs regarding scope of practice are more apparent.

There appears to be a growing divergence in the general direction of NP versus PA practice patterns. Perhaps as many as three-fourths of America's 27,000 NPs work in primary care. NPs practice mainly in the areas of adult medicine, pediatrics, women's health, student health, and geriatrics.[37] In contrast, while PAs continue to practice in primary care and hold strong potential to expand medical service delivery in needy settings, they have fulfilled this potential only to a modest degree, particularly in rural and medically underserved areas, where both PA and physician numbers in recent years have fallen.[38] Evidently emulating physician practice patterns, PAs are increasingly drawn to specialty settings and acute care roles.[39] Expanded demand for PAs in GME resident substitution positions accentuates this trend, further splitting both policy objectives and the PA profession itself between the traditional primary care role and specialty practice. NPs, on the other hand, remain employed mostly in primary care and seem likely to develop expanded roles as care givers in nursing homes, home care, and community-based settings.[40]

Other health professionals may vie for opportunities to provide primary care to populations in medical shortage areas. For several decades, cross-linkages have existed between the roles and professional relationships of PAs and international medical graduates. Beginning in the mid-1970s, after more than 20 years of an open-door policy in U.S. medical education, immigration laws pertaining to IMG entry tightened. Many large, urban teaching hospitals depended upon IMGs to meet personnel requirements in GME programs and clinical inpatient staffing. The decreased IMG supply increased demand for PAs to assume house staff and resident substitute roles.

Throughout the 1980s, as residency programs and teaching services adjusted medical staff size and configuration, PAs increasingly assumed inpatient care roles formerly held by IMGs. Recently, unlicensed IMGs in several states have attempted to obtain qualification to work as PAs, arguing that as PAs they can work in the health occupation for which they were trained and deliver services in medically needy areas. PAs have opposed such moves, citing the differences in role orientation between dependent and independent providers and potential confusion if IMGs are cast as PAs.

Who Will Provide Primary Care?

It may be unrealistic to expect that physicians will by themselves reverse trends of professional specialization. Established specialists are unlikely to convert to generalist roles. The continuing decline in interest among young physicians in primary care careers and generalist practice is painfully apparent.[41] Even if the number of medical graduates choosing primary care significantly increases, decades would pass before adjustments in graduate medical education outcomes will have an impact on service delivery.

As physicians become increasingly specialized, non-physician health providers are likely to assume a greater profile in delivering primary care. This prospect is particularly likely in health maintenance organizations, other types of managed care systems and organized health care systems such as VA, state and federal correctional systems, and the military. Some feel that physicians are really no longer in the primary care business and that PAs, working with physician "managers," may be the providers best equipped to meet future primary care needs. These people are recommending increased PA educational output and utilization in primary care roles.[42]

Any health care workforce strategy to reduce costs and increase access must take maximal advantage of the practice competencies of non-physicians. Restructuring the health care system to deliver the bulk of primary care through PAs and NPs and having physicians assume increased management and consulting duties would likely be more economical for many institutions and would better utilize medical training and talent. Non-physician providers may be better suited than physicians to performing certain clinical functions, such as counseling, chronic disease management, and preventive care.[43]

The future for PAs and other non-physician health professionals will likely be determined by political, economic, and legal factors affecting the evolution of their roles in relation to those of physicians. As our health care system changes from a disease-oriented and economically open-ended structure to a more preventive, patient-centered, cost-conscious one, non-physicians will assume a higher profile. The further evolution of the professional roles of PAs and other non-physicians in U.S. health care will be determined by changing trends in the division of medical labor — trends that reflect public percep-tions of physician responsiveness to patient needs and that better serve the public interest.[44] Under scenarios considering future de-mands for health services, providers with a primary care or generalist orientation will markedly increase, particularly if some form of uni-versal health coverage is implemented.[45]

The Need for Increased Research

Research on the clinical and professional activities of PAs and other non-physician providers has languished in recent years, following extensive investigations conducted in the 1970s. While much is known from this research and widespread experience with PAs, many aspects of PAs' clinical roles and contributions remain poorly under-stood. What is the optimal mix of health care providers to deliver primary care? How can the economic advantages of these providers be best used in health systems of the future? How many PAs, NPs, physicians, and other health professionals will be needed to staff emerging types of managed care systems and meet anticipated health workforce needs in primary care and GME-related areas?

Planning should commence to assess America's present health care workforce capacities, to consider short- and long-term population-based need for medical services, and to articulate these concerns with national goals for health status.[46] The general lack of accurate information on non-physician activities in the health workforce places policy makers at a disadvantage in attempts to promote more effective use of PAs and to better coordinate their supply and utilization with physicians.

Research concerning non-physician practice should center on:
- Determination of maximal physician substitution potentials, the optimal effectiveness of using PAs in GME positions, and the impact of such changes on teaching hospitals and resi-dency programs.
- Description of current practice characteristics and content of care delivered by PAs in primary care, including clinical pre-ventive services; measurement of PA clinical productivity and patient care outcomes in various settings.

- Description of the economic aspects of PA practice, including revenue generation, practice costs, potential for savings, and optimal staffing mix.

Recommendations

The following recommendations aim to increase the contribution of PAs in addressing current medical workforce issues and augment efficiency in medical care.

1) Increase PA supply by expanding PA educational program output with an annual goal of 3,500 to 4,000 PA graduates by 2000.

- Increase Title VII funding for the Grants Program for PA education with the objective of expanding the production of PA health personnel.
- Include through grant programs incentives to increase enrollment capacities in existing programs and support the development of new PA educational programs set in academic health centers, colleges, and universities.
- Provide continued incentives for PA education programs to emphasize primary care and include rewards for PA programs that effectively deploy graduates in rural and medically underserved areas.
- Increase training capabilities in PA programs considering anticipated roles in hospital-based settings and GME programs.
- Link Medicare GME support to fund clinical educational experiences for PA students in teaching hospitals, and offer incentives for PA training and establishing PA programs in academic health centers.
- Encourage academic health centers preparing to reduce undergraduate or graduate medical education programs to sponsor PA training programs or expand affiliations and clinical teaching activities supporting the increased production of PAs.

2) Lower barriers to PA clinical effectiveness.

- Authorize Medicare Part B reimbursement for PA clinical services delivered in outpatient and ambulatory settings.
- Permit off-site supervision in both urban and rural settings.
- Encourage state Medicaid programs to cover medical care services rendered by PAs, and discourage states from discounting payments.

- Increase the Medicare bonus paid to clinical practices employing non-physicians in primary care settings in underserved areas.
- Encourage state medical licensing boards to modify PA scope-of-practice and prescribing laws to allow for the attainment of maximal utilization potentials of these health providers.

3) Include PAs and NPs in future health care workforce planning.

- If a national health care workforce planning commission is constituted, this body should coordinate health professions education and utilization activities so that the practice advantages of PAs and NPs are incorporated with roles of other health care professionals to improve efficiency and social responsiveness in medical care services delivery.
- Make expanded research funding available to examine PA and NP capabilities, clinical and economic performance in various settings, and potentials for utilization in future health services systems.

References

1. Health Resources and Services Administration, Council on Graduate Medical Education. Improving Access to Health Care Through Physician Workforce Reform. Rockville, Md: US Government Printing Office; 1992.
2. United States Congress, Office of Technology Assessment. *Nurse Practitioners, Physician Assistants, and Certified Nurse-Midwives: A Policy Analysis.* Health Care Technology Case Study No. 37. Washington, DC: National Technical Information Service; 1986. Record JC, McCally ME, Schwietzer SO, et al. New health professionals after a decade and a half: delegation, productivity, and costs in primary care. *J Health Politics Policy Law.* 1980;5:470-497. Schafft GE, Cawley JF. *Physician Assistants in a Changing Health Care Environment.* Rockville, Md: Aspen Publishers; 1987.
3. Health Resources and Services Administration, Bureau of Health Professions. *Health Personnel in the United States: Eighth Report to Congress 1991.* Rockville, Md: US Government Printing Office; 1992.
4. Weiner JP, Steinwachs DM, Williamson JW. Nurse practitioner and physician assistant practices in three HMOs: implications for future US health manpower needs. *Am J Pub Health.* 1986;76:507-511. Starfield B. *Primary Care: Concept, Evaluation, and Policy.* New York: Oxford University Press; 1992.
5. Record JC, McCally ME, Schwietzer SO, et al. New health professionals after a decade and a half: delegation, productivity, and costs in primary care. *J Health Politics Policy Law.* 1980;5:470-497.
6. United States Congress, Office of Technology Assessment. *Nurse Practitioners, Physician Assistants, and Certified Nurse-Midwives: A Policy Analysis.* Health Care Technology Case Study No. 37. Washington, DC: National Technical Information Service; 1986. Weiner JP, Steinwachs DM, Williamson JW. Nurse practitioner and physician assistant practices in three HMOs: implications for future US health manpower needs. *Am J Pub Health.* 1986;76:507-511. Johnson RE, Freeborn DK, McCally M. Delegation of office visits in primary care to PAs and NPs: the physicians' view. *Physician Assistant.* 1985;5:159-169.
7. Alexander BJ, Lipscomb, J. Nonphysician panel report. In: Institute of Medicine. *Physician Staffing for the VA.* Volume II. Alexandria, Va: National Academy Press; 1992.
8. McGill F, Kliener GJ, Vanderbilt C, et al. Postgraduate internship in gynecology and obstetrics for physician assistants: a four-year experience. *Obstetrics and Gynecology.* 1990;76:1135-1139.

9. Cawley JF. *The Cost Effectiveness of Physician Assistants.* Alexandria, VA: American Academy of Physician Assistants; 1986.

10. Zarbock SF, Harbert K, eds. *Physician Assistants: Present and Future Models of Utilization.* New York: Praeger Publishers; 1986.

11. Asch DA, Ende J. The downsizing of internal medicine residency programs. *Ann Int Med.* 1992;117:839-844.

12. Heinrich JJ, Fichandler BC, Krizik TS, et al. The physician assistant as resident on surgical services. *Archives Surg.* 1980;115:310-314.

13. McKelvey PA, Oliver DA, Conboy JE. PA roles in a tertiary medical center. *Physician Assistant.* 1986;10:149-159.

14. Demots H, Coombs B, Murphy E, Palac D. Coronary arteriography performed by a physician assistant. *Am J Cardiology.* 1987;60:784-787.

15. Dubaybo BA, Samson MK, Carlson RW. The role of the physician assistant in critical care units. *Chest.* 1991;99:89-91.

16. Asch DA, Ende J. The downsizing of internal medicine.

17. Lieberman DA, Ghormley JM. Physician assistants in gastroenterology: should they perform endoscopy? *Am J Gastroent.* 1992;87:940-943.

18. Schafft GE, Cawley JF. *Physician Assistants in a Changing Health Care Environment.* Rockville, Md: Aspen Publishers; 1987.

19. Hooker RS. *The Role of Physician Assistants and Nurse Practitioners in a Managed Care Setting.* Washington, DC: Association of Academic Health Centers; 1993.

20. Eastaugh SE. Hospital nursing technical efficiency: nurse extenders and enhanced productivity. *Hosp Health Serv Admin.* 1990;35:561-573.

21. Nichols LM. Estimating costs of underusing advanced practice nurses. *Nursing Economics.* 1992;10:343-351.

22. Health Resources and Services Administration, Bureau of Health Professions. *Health Personnel in the United States: Eighth Report to Congress 1991.* Rockville, Md: US Government Printing Office; 1992.

23. *Annual Census Data on Physician Assistants, 1992.* Alexandria, Va: American Academy of Physician Assistants; 1992.

24. Cawley JF. Hospital physician assistants: past, present, and future. *Hospital Topics.* 1991;61:9-14.

25. Willis JB, Pylitt LL. Physician assistants and hospital practice. *J Am Acad Phys Asst.* 1993;6:115-122.

26. *Annual Census Data on Physician Assistants, 1992.* Alexandria, Va: American Academy of Physician Assistants; 1992.

27. Oliver DR. *Eighth Annual Report on Physician Assistant Educational Programs in the United States, 1991-1992.* Alexandria, Va: Association of Physician Assistant Programs; 1992.

28. Health Resources and Services Administration, Bureau of Health Professions. *Health Personnel in the United States: Eighth Report to Congress 1991.* Rockville, Md: US Government Printing Office; 1992.

29. *Annual Census Data on Physician Assistants, 1992.* Alexandria, Va: American Academy of Physician Assistants; 1992.

30. Oliver DR. *Eighth Annual Report on Physician Assistant Educational Programs.*

31. Alexander BJ, Lipscomb, J. Nonphysician panel report. In: Institute of Medicine. *Physician Staffing for the VA.* Volume II. Alexandria, Va: National Academy Press; 1992.

32. Silver HK, McAtee PA. On the use of nonphysician "associate residents" in overcrowded specialty-training programs. *New Eng J Med.* 1984;311:326-328.

33. Mullan F. Missing: a national medical manpower policy. *Milbank Fund Q.* 1992;70:381-386.

34. Thorpe KE. House staff supervision and working hours: implications of regulatory change in New York State. *JAMA.* 1990;263:3177-3181.

35. Asch DA, Ende J. The downsizing of internal medicine residency programs. *Ann Int Med.* 1992;117:839-844.

36. Knickman JR, Lipkin M, Finkler SA, Thompson WG, Kiel J. The potential for using non-physicians to compensate for the reduced availability of residents. *Academic Med.* 1992;67:429-438.

37. Harper, Doreen. Personal communication. George Mason University; February, 1993.

38. United States Congress, Office of Technology Assessment. Problems in the recruitment and retention of rural health personnel. In: *Health Care in Rural America.* Washington, DC: US Government Printing Office; 1990. Publication OTA-H-434.

39. Hooker RS. Employment specialization in the PA profession. *J Am Acad Phys Asst.* 1992;5:695-704.

40. Evarts CM, Bosomworth PP, Osterweis M, eds. *Human Resources for Health: Defining the Future.* Washington, DC: Association of Academic Health Centers; 1992.

41. Colwill JM. Where have all the primary care applicants gone? *New Eng J Med.* 1992;326:387-394.

42. Miekle T. An expanded role for the physician assistant. *Bellwether.* Vol.3, No.3, 1992.

43. United States Congress, Office of Technology Assessment. *Nurse Practitioners, Physician Assistants, and Certified Nurse-Midwives: A Policy Analysis.* Health Care Technology Case Study No. 37. Washington, DC: National Technical Information Service; 1986.

44. Fryer GE. The United States medical profession: an abnormal form of the division of labor. *Sociology Health Illness.* 1991;13:213-230.

45. Weiner J. The effects of future health care system trends on the demand for physician services: an assessment of selected specialties. Prepared for the Council on Graduate Medical Education. Rockville, Md: Health Resources and Services Administration, #91-406P; 1991.

46. Mullan F. Missing: a national medical manpower policy. *Milbank Fund Q.* 1992;70:381-386.

4

Nurse Practitioners: Educational Issues, Practice Styles, and Service Barriers

Sheila A. Ryan

FOR THREE DECADES, NURSE PRACTITIONERS (NPs), certified nurse midwives (CNMs), and other nurses with advanced education and practice skills have provided primary health care to the nation. Considerable research has been generated on these providers' acceptability, cost-effectiveness, and substitutability for physicians in the provision of primary care.

Because primary care is seen as dealing with mundane, everyday health care concerns rather than high technology or life-and-death diseases, it has long been undervalued by policy makers.[1] Consideration of national health reform offers an excellent opportunity to redesign policies, delivery systems and research support for primary care.

Educational Preparation and Titling Issues

While there are three main categories of advanced nurse practitioners, other certified specialty nurses create titling issues that require some clarification. Advanced NPs complete advanced study, usually at the graduate level, and are certified by state authorities for advanced or expanded practice. Most hold national certification by exam from the American Nurses Association (ANA) or other national organizations. Their titles include adult nurse practitioner, family nurse practitioner, pediatric nurse practitioner, gerontological nurse practitioner, school nurse practitioner, and women's health nurse practitioner.

The majority of care provided by NPs is primary care. It is estimated that 60 percent to 90 percent of ambulatory primary care can be effectively managed by NPs.[2] Recently, a trend has begun emerging to prepare and use acute care and neonatal intensive care nurse practitioners for hospital residency substitution.

Currently, there are approximately 20,000 certified NPs whose advanced practice privileges include prescriptive authority in 37 states. In addition, there are 5,000 certified nurse midwives and 28,000 certified nurse anesthetists. There are also clinical nurse specialists — advanced practice nurses in a specialty area of graduate study who usually practice in hospital roles providing indirect care. Examples include oncology nurse specialists, cardiovascular nurse specialists, and psychiatric and mental health nurse specialists.

Further, there are specialty nurses who are certified by their specialty organization but whose preparation does not include formal graduate study. Examples are enterostomal nurses, diabetes educators, nephrology and dialysis nurses, orthopedic nurses, rehabilitation nurses, infection control nurses, emergency nurses, and perioperative nurses. This category totals approximately 190,600 nurses but is not included in the advanced practice/nurse practitioner discussion.

Studies have shown that the direct costs of education for NPs are approximately one-fifth of those for physicians. The congressional Office of Technology Assessment (OTA) estimated that in 1985 the costs approximated $86,100 for physicians, $14,600 for NPs, and $16,800 for CNMs.[3] Thus, several NPs could be trained for the cost of educating one physician. Most NP and CNM programs can be completed in a two-year, post-baccalaureate program. The costs are defrayed primarily by the government in the form of subsidized tuition, grants and loans to students, and grants to educational institutions for clinical training and research.

Safriet concludes that regardless of the current and true costs, total physician training costs, both direct and indirect, are clearly at least four to five times greater than those for NPs and CNMs.[4]

Recently, the University of Rochester initiated a post-graduate practitioner preparation course for clinical nurse specialists (CNSs) interested in qualifying for nurse practitioner certification. This program consists of advanced primary health care skills, assessment, and pharmacology study. Students can complete the course within a year while working full time. The course has been well received by CNS nurses (40 students are currently enrolled).

With moderate educational incentives and stimuli, nursing programs could double the number of primary care practitioners by the end of this decade.

Clinical Effectiveness

A study requested by the United States Congress and conducted by the OTA in 1986 concluded that the care of these various nurse providers is of equivalent quality to that provided by physicians.[5] A study of 248 documents on NP effectiveness conducted by Feldman, Ventura, and Crosby reported consistent findings with that of the OTA study.[6] The findings indicate that patients are satisfied, that nurses' interpersonal skills are better than those of physicians, that the technical quality of their services is equivalent, that patient outcomes are equivalent or superior to those effected by physicians, and that nurses facilitate continuity of patient care as well as improved access to care in underserved areas.

A third study, a meta-analysis of process of care, clinical outcomes, and cost-effectiveness of nurse practitioners and nurse midwives in primary care roles, was reported in December 1992.[7] NPs provided more health promotion activities and scored higher on quality-of-care measures than did physicians. NPs ordered more laboratory tests, though these tests were less costly. The average cost per laboratory test was $20.49 for NP patients and $22.36 for physician's patients, an 8 percent savings for NP patients over MD patients.

Drug prescription rates and patient knowledge were both equivalent. And NPs achieved higher scores than physicians on issues of patient satisfaction, patient compliance, pathological resolution, and functional status.[8]

Nurses spent 24.9 minutes per patient, on average, and physicians spent 16.5 minutes. The number of visits per patient was equivalent for both provider groups; however, the NP patients experienced fewer hospitalizations than did physician patients. The average cost per NP visit was $12.36, compared with $20.11 for physician patients. (This finding acknowledges clear confounding of regional and salary differentials.)

Critics of NP/CNM research have suggested that the variation in outcomes of care may result from physicians' patients being sicker than NPs' patients. In the study referred to above, the investigators attempted control for client risk differentials by calculating effect sizes on categorical model-testing but were unable to conduct such an analysis because of too few effect sizes per cell. Consequently, they used only randomized study trials where subjects to provider groups had been controlled for process, client, and setting differences. Outcome data compared low-risk patients only. When data from experimental studies only were re-analyzed separately with patient risk controlled, results either did not change or NP groups produced more favorable results.

CNM practices differed from physician practices in that they used less analgesia and anesthesia, performed less fetal monitoring, did fewer episiotomies, forceps deliveries and amniotomies, and administered less intravenous fluids. CNMs induced labor less frequently, but their patients had equivalent rates of Caesarean sections.

Infant clinical outcomes (fetal distress, one-minute Apgar scores, and low birthweight) and neonatal mortality rates were equivalent for CNMs and MDs. CNM patients achieved higher five-minute Apgar scores and experienced more spontaneous vaginal deliveries than did MD patients. Fifty-three percent of CNM patients breast-fed their infants, compared to 24 percent of MD patients. The mean percentage of low birthweight babies was 6.5 percent for CNM patients and 7.4 percent for MD patients. The average rates of prematurity were 4.5 percent for CNM patients and 10 percent for physician patients. The mean length of hospital stay was 2.1 days for CNM patients and 2.9 days for physician patients. CNM patients had more prenatal and postpartum visits than did MD patients.[9] The CNM/MD comparison studies did not control for patient risk.

Given that NP and CNM patient outcomes are equivalent to, or better than, those of physicians, the lower costs associated with educating and employing NPs and CNMs result in the cost-effective provision of quality primary care services. Although the expanded roles for NPs and CNMs were originally designed for rural areas and underserved populations, most of the research was conducted in urban areas.

The studies repeatedly affirm that NPs and CNMs, in a wide variety of settings, can substantially increase access to high quality basic health care for people who would have been otherwise underserved. These findings are not remarkable, according to Safriet.

What is remarkable is that these providers have been able to achieve these results despite multiple legal and professional restrictions on their practice.[10]

Issues in Research and Reimbursement

Much more research is needed regarding the care provided by NPs and MDs, especially in processes of care, cost-effectiveness, and outcomes, such as quality of life, functional status, and illness avoidance. Research must be encouraged to determine the most cost-effective mix of nurses and physician providers in various practice settings, in emerging delivery systems, and with different populations.

Measuring the employment costs of NPs and CNMs against physicians is both simple and complicated. Salaries, office costs, and support staff are easy to measure, yet the provider groups differ in the process and content of care they provide.

Several studies have concluded that advanced non-physician providers are seriously underutilized in today's health care system.[11] The reasons for this underuse are many and controversial. They include legal scope-of-practice restrictions, delegation, supervision and reimbursement policies, and size of training programs. For example, NPs and CNMs use high-technology diagnostic and therapeutic measures less frequently than do physicians; this behavior could affect total practice revenue or at least per-procedure utilization.

It is also difficult to measure the effects upon practice revenues of non-physician providers' emphasis on wellness and prevention. While society would clearly benefit from reduction in illness, the effects could be perceived as detrimental to the employers in a cost-reimbursed delivery system. In a competitive, managed arena, such behavior would be perceived as valuable. Until physician and provider fees are fully regulated within a managed competition system, fee-for-service should use the Resource-Based Relative Value Scale, with relative weights favoring primary care services.[12]

Medicare's Graduate Medical Education (GME) payments can also increase the utilization of advanced non-physician providers. The stated rationale of these payments is to compensate for costs borne by educational programs that are not paid for by patient care revenues. GME payments should be made to advanced health professionals whose training provides primary care services, should strengthen incentives for primary care provider residencies, and should include non-hospital training sites, such as ambulatory care and health centers, whether they are "teaching" or "non-teaching" by classification. Hospitals receive GME payment when their residents rotate through primary care sites, but the sites are not paid directly for their own trainees.

Overall, policy makers must put more money toward primary care. General funding for primary care programs, such as migrant health, family planning, Preventative Health Block grant, and Maternal and Child Health Block grant, have remained level or shown small increases, rising to $480 million in 1991.[13] This figure pales in comparison to $8.3 billion from Medicare payments to hospitals for capital-related payments in FY 1993. And a recent estimate suggested that $40 million from the federal government was available for primary care research, while NIH funding is $10.4 billion.

Barriers to Service

Barriers that impede the efficient and effective delivery of basic health care include a health care system that imposes numerous limitations on patients and would-be patients seeking care. Restrictive state provisions governing scope of practice and prescriptive authority, as well as fragmented state and federal standards for reimbursement, severely hamper the ability of NPs and CNMs to fulfill their proven potential to enhance our nation's health.

Effective changes within the health delivery system that promote primary care services are second in the health reform debate to funding strategies.[14] Managed care systems must be structured to ensure that case managers are primary care practitioners instead of insurance clerks and to favor hospital-physician groups that reduce the number of specialists.

If health insurance purchasing cooperatives become the method of managed competition, reform, and payment, then salaried physicians, NPs, and PAs alike will be contracted through hospitals to help provide cost-effective basic health care and produce quality care outcomes.

Nurse practitioners have added value over primary care MDs or PAs because of the nursing profession's ability to produce a rapid supply of primary care practitioners already being educated to serve populations, with emphasis on primary care, preventive care, community care, and health promotion.[15]

Conclusion

Safriet[16] summarizes these issues well:

> The potential of advanced practice nurses to increase access to good care at a reasonable cost is nicely summarized in a 1991 study[17] of physician and NP clinical decision making. The providers, drawn from a stratified random sample of internists, family practitioners, and general practitioners listed in the AMA census files and from a list provided by the American Academy of Nurse Practitioners, included 501 physicians and 298 NPs. During telephone interviews, these practitioners were presented with the following case vignette of a patient with abdominal pain:
>
>> A man you have never seen before comes to your office seeking help for intermittent sharp epigastric pains that are relieved by meals but are worse on an empty stomach. The patient has just moved from out of state and brings along a report of an endoscopy performed a month ago showing diffuse gastritis of moderate severity, but no ulcer. Is there a particular therapy you would choose at this point, or would you need additional information?[18]

During the interviews, participants were repeatedly asked if there was any additional patient information they would want before formulating a treatment plan. If they asked, standardized responses to questions revealed the following:

> medications currently used: two aspirin tablets four times daily for stomach pain; social or psychological history: the patient's son was killed in a car accident eight weeks ago; diet: five cups of coffee per day, one large meal (at lunch); smoking: two packs per day; alcohol: two cocktails with lunch and two glasses of wine in the evening; and other previous medical history and review of systems: unremarkable.

As noted in the study results,

> "striking differences were found in the diagnostic and therapeutic style of nurse practitioners when compared with physicians."[19] For example, twice as many physicians as NPs chose to initiate treatment without seeking any additional information about the patient. When additional information was sought, NPs were "far more likely to ask about the patient's diet and psychosocial situation." When a therapeutic intervention was proposed, 63 percent of the physicians opted to write a prescription, whereas only 20 percent of the NPs chose to do so. Rather, the NPs more often recommended "a change in diet or counseling to help the patient deal with stress. . .which would have been more appropriate in the case of a patient with gastritis and high aspirin, caffeine,

alcohol, and tobacco intake."[20]

The fact that "Far more nurses than physicians elicited the basic historical information necessary to make an intelligent treatment plan for the patients presented" has inescapable implications for both the quality of care and its cost. As the study authors observed, many have argued that the health care system must find a way to provide reimbursement for the time spent in history taking and patient counseling. While this is probably true, it is interesting to note that in this instance nurse practitioners, who are reimbursed at a lower level, appear to have performed these tasks more completely.[21]

This study captures, in a nutshell, both the promise of advanced practice nursing, as well as the shortcomings of the present health care delivery system. Much of that promise can be realized if state and federal governments implement the specific proposals enumerated above. Especially if they understand and embrace the vision of advanced practice nursing that animates these proposals, they will effectively carry out their mandate to protect the public and enhance the availability of high quality, cost-effective health services. APNs (advanced practice nurses) are proven providers; removing the many barriers to their practice will only increase their ability to respond to the pressing need for basic health care in our country.

References

1. Budetti P. Achieving a uniform federal primary care policy: opportunities presented by national health reform. *JAMA*. 1993;269:498-501.

2. Brown SA, Grimes DE. *Nurse Practitioners and Certified Nurse Midwives: A Meta-Analysis of Studies on Nurses in Primary Care Roles*. Washington, DC: American Nurses Association; March, 1993.

3. United States Congress, Office of Technology Assessment. *Nurse Practitioners, Physician Assistants, and Certified Nurse-Midwives: A Policy Analysis*. Washington, DC: U.S. Government Printing Office; 1986. Health Technology Case Study 37, OTA-HCS-37.

4. Safriet BJ. Health care dollars and regulatory sense: the role of advanced practice nursing. *Yale J Regulation*. 1992;9(2): 417-488.

5. United States Congress. Office of Technology Assessment. *Nurse Practitioners, Physician Assistants, and Certified Nurse-Midwives: A Policy Analysis*. Washington, DC: U.S. Government Printing Office; 1986. Health Technology Case Study 37, OTA-HCS-37.

6. Feldman MJ, Ventura MR, Crosby F. Studies of nurse practitioners effectiveness. *Nursing Research.* 1987;36:303-8.

7. Brown SA, Grimes, DE. Nurse Practitioners and Certified Nurse Midwives: *A Meta-Analysis of Studies on Nurses in Primary Care Roles.* Washington, DC: American Nurses Association; March, 1993.

8. Hall J, Palmer H, Orau J, et al. Performance, quality, gender and professional role: a study of physicians and non-physicians in 16 ambulatory care practices. *Medical Care.* 1990;28:489-501.

9. Graveley E, Littlefield J. A cost-effectiveness analysis of three staffing models in the delivery of low risk prenatal care. *Am J Public Health.* 1992;82:180-184.

10. Safriet BJ. Health care dollars and regulatory sense: the role of advanced practice nursing. *Yale J Regulation.* 1992;9(2): 417-488.

11. Nichols LM. Estimating costs of underusing advanced practice nurses. *Nursing Economics.* 1992;10:343-351.

12. Budetti P. Achieving a uniform federal primary care policy: opportunities presented by national health reform. *JAMA.* 1993;269:498-501.

13. Budetti, P. Achieving a uniform federal primary care policy: opportunities presented by national health reform. *JAMA.* 1993;269:498-501.
14. O'Neil EH. *Health Professions Education for the Future: Schools in Service to the Nation.* San Francisco, Calif: Pew Health Professions Commission; 1993.
15. American Nurses Association. *Nursing's Agenda For Health Care Reform.* Washington, DC: American Nurses Association; 1991.
16. Safriet BJ. Health care dollars and regulatory sense: the role of advanced practice nursing. *Yale J Regulation.* 1992; 9 (2): 417-488.
17. Avorn J, Everitt DE, Baker MW. The neglected medical history and therapeutic choices for abdominal pain: a nationwide study of 799 physicians and nurses. *Arch Intern Med.* 1991;151:694-698 in Safriet BJ. Health care dollars and regulatory sense. *Yale J Regulation.* 1992; 9(2):417-488.
18. Avorn J, Everitt DE, Baker MW. The neglected medical history and therapeutic choices for abdominal pain: a nationwide study of 799 physicians and nurses. *Arch Intern Med.* 1991;151:694-698 in Safriet BJ. Health care dollars and regulatory sense. *Yale J Regulation.* 1992; 9(2):417-488.
19. Avorn J, Everitt DE, Baker MW. The neglected medical history and therapeutic choices for abdominal pain: a nationwide study of 799 physicians and nurses. *Arch Intern Med.* 1991;151:694-698 in Safriet BJ. Health care dollars and regulatory sense. *Yale J Regulation.* 1992; 9(2):417-488.
20. Avorn J, Everitt DE, Baker MW. The neglected medical history and therapeutic choices for abdominal pain: a nationwide study of 799 physicians and nurses. *Arch Intern Med.* 1991;151:694-698 in Safriet BJ. Health care dollars and regulatory sense. *Yale J Regulation.* 1992; 9(2):417-488.
21. Avorn J, Everitt DE, Baker MW. The neglected medical history and therapeutic choices for abdominal pain: a nationwide study of 799 physicians and nurses. *Arch Intern Med.* 1991;151:694-698 in Safriet BJ. Health care dollars and regulatory sense. *Yale J Regulation.* 1992; 9(2):417-488.

5

The Roles of Physician Assistants and Nurse Practitioners in a Managed Care Organization

Roderick S. Hooker

W IDE VARIATIONS EXIST ACROSS COMMUNITIES and organizations in the use of medical services and personnel. Not only do the types of health manpower employed in physician offices vary, but quality differences among these types affect their relative productivities. Based on the literature, it appears that physician assistants (PAs) and pediatric nurse practitioners (PNPs) are the closest substitutes for physicians in the primary care outpatient setting, and nurse anesthetists (CRNAs) for anesthesiologists as specialists in the inpatient setting.

But what fraction of a physician can PAs and NPs replace, and how many are needed to replace that physician fraction? This paper examines the collaborative practice of primary care physicians, PAs and NPs in one type of health care setting that has accumulated more than two decades of experience with non-physician providers.

Background

In 1970, the Kaiser Permanente Northwest Region (KPNW) became the first non-academic institution to hire both a formally trained PA and a PNP. KPNW hired them not to fill specific vacancies but to gain experience for future staffing needs.[1] KPNW had previous experience with other types of non-physician professionals: optometrists, nurse anesthetists, nurse midwives, and psychologists.[2] KPNW believed that a PA and an NP could be useful adjuncts to the primary care physician in a large group practice.

KPNW soon recognized that the PA and NP were not only functioning effectively in this capacity but could be used for more advanced roles than originally envisioned. The PA could provide needed manpower and skills in trauma management, refill prescriptions, and assume the care of many chronic conditions, such as diabetes, hypertension, and atherosclerotic heart disease. The PNP could handle routine care, such as well-baby checks, parent education, and immunizations, and also manage common pediatric problems, such as upper respiratory infections, otitis media, and dermatitis.

Within 10 years, eight departments had incorporated a PA or NP, and the tasks these non-physicians were performing, as well as the types of ambulatory patients they were seeing, differed little from their physician counterparts in the same outpatient department setting.[3] They saw a similar number of patients daily and exceeded physicians' annual patient visit rates because they maintained an exclusively ambulatory care role, occupying an office more often and with less compensatory time off than physicians.

A number of studies have attempted to estimate the best use of PAs and NPs in physician practices. One study used activity analysis to model the optimal organization of a primary care practice.[4] It listed 263 tasks that fully describe most typical primary care practices, developed a model and estimated that introducing a PA would increase productivity by 49 to 74 percent. That is, a physician usually producing 147 office visits per week might increase that number to 265 visits per week simply by hiring a PA.

Reinhardt concluded that physicians in groups generate between 4.5 and 5.1 percent more patient visits and about 5.6 percent more patient billings than those in solo practice.[5] These results suggest slight economies of scale. Reinhardt also found that productivity of physicians increased with group size because of greater manpower substitution in groups.[6]

Evidence indicates that organizational setting is related to the productivity and possible cost benefits of PAs. Scheffler documents that PAs in institutions are more productive than PAs in private practice; they see more patients in the same period.[7] Noting a correlation between productivity, task delegation, and organizational size, Record and colleagues offer economies of scale and incentives for cost containment as plausible explanations. They also estimate that if enough PAs were hired to perform all of the services for which they are considered competent, and if PA and MD workweeks were equated, the substitution ratio would be .76.[8] Page's data, developed in the military, led him to suggest a ratio closer to unity (1:1).[9] In 1986, it was found that the number of patients (with similar presenting morbidities) seen per hour and per day by PAs and physicians in a health maintenance organization's departments of internal medicine and family practice were almost the same.[10] Overall, it seems that the theoretical estimates of PA productivity are higher in large managed care organizations, such as health maintenance organizations and the military, with controversy centering on estimates of productivity in solo practice.[11]

During the past 15 years, various social and economic trends have shifted the center of direction for medical care from community hospitals to managed health care systems. One form of managed care that has received a lot of attention is the prepaid group practice, or health maintenance organization (HMO). Utilization of PAs and NPs in these settings has not gone unnoticed by health systems managers in managed medical care organizations.

The Setting
KPNW is a large, group-model HMO located in Portland, Oregon, that provides comprehensive medical care to approximately 380,000 members. In 1992, 520 full-time equivalent (FTE) physicians (540 actual) represented all major and most minor subspecialties.[12] Because KPNW is a comprehensive health and medical plan, it employs a wide variety of providers to deliver general and technical care (see Figure 1). These providers manage approximately 2.5 million patient encounters each year. Members choose one of 17 medical offices for primary or specialty care and two Kaiser hospitals. KPNW is unique in that it has a prepaid dental HMO component as well.

Adult primary care is organized by the departments of internal medicine and family practice. Each department is composed of physicians, PAs, and NPs. Each department, depending on its office layout, includes modules of five to seven clinicians. A typical module may contain four physicians, a PA, and an NP, constituting a shared practice. Within this module, the providers determine how patients are managed, depending on demands for care and certain provider

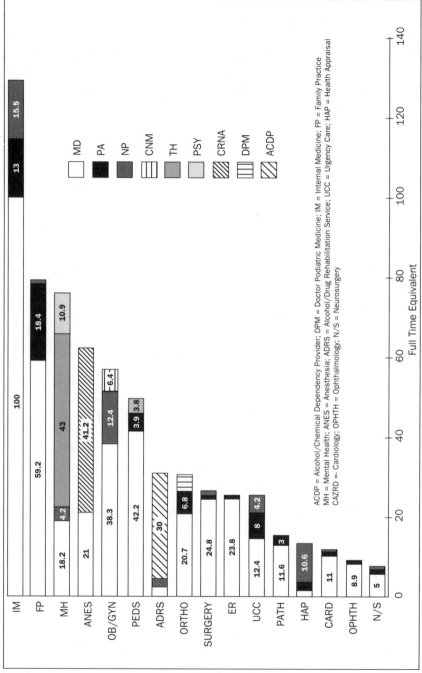

Figure 1
Kaiser Permanente Northwest Region Provider Staffing (FTE) 1992

inclinations. For example, one internist may have a youthful panel of members who have selected him as a primary care provider, but he will ask them to see the NP for annual pelvic screening examinations. On the other hand, the PA may have an interest in diabetes care and, through agreement with her module and the module nurse coordinator, may shift diabetic patients to her practice for chronic management.

Each module has certain styles and practice arrangements, but all are established to manage most primary care conditions. Usually, all providers in a module share urgent and non-appointment cases and serve as "gatekeepers." In order to avoid unduly burdening clinicians with elderly patients and complex cases, each physician's panel is weighted by a formula that is assigned according to age group. Thus, if a physician has a practice skewed to the elderly, the panel size is kept smaller than average. When a physician's panel is full, his or her practice is closed to new members until member turnover allows it to be reopened. Unassigned members, people who are new to the health plan as well as those who do not want a primary care provider, are usually given an appointment with the first available provider.

Determination of the type of provider is at the discretion of the chief of service. In the primary care area of family practice, PAs make up one-third of the contingent; in internal medicine, one-fifth; the urgency care clinic is evenly divided among physicians and PAs/NPs; and the health appraisal program is run almost exclusively by NPs. In fact, the administrative head of the health appraisal program is an NP, and that of the urgency care clinic is a PA.

Table 1 lists some of the expanding roles of PAs and NPs. However, staffing appears to be largely a function of physician attitudes, and determined by the physician group.[13] For instance, KPNW general surgeons have largely relied on resident house officers and technicians instead of PAs to assist in surgery, in spite of the high use of PAs in neurosurgery and orthopedics. Ironically, across the nation, 25 percent of all graduate PAs are in a surgical specialty or subspecialty.[14] Furthermore, the various Kaiser Permanente regions differ markedly in their use of PAs and NPs. The Northern California region employs a handful of PAs but 360 NPs, while the Southern California region has more than 500 PAs and NPs on staff.

Table 1
The Roles of PAs and NPs in KPNW

Administration	Neurosurgery
Alcohol/Chemical	OB/Gyn
Cardiology	Ophthalmology
Dermatology	Orthopedics
Endocrinology	Pathology
Emergency Medicine	Pediatrics
Family Practice	Psychiatry
Gastroenterology	Research
Gerontology	Rheumatology
Internal Medicine	Urgency Care
Mental Health	

Productivity

"In theory, productivity is a simple concept — it measures changes in total output that occur when small changes are made in one factor of production, with all other factors and circumstances held constant. Because these conditions can be met in the real world only rarely, productivity numbers are almost always rough estimates with respect to physicians."[15]

What happens to the output of a physician's practice when a PA or NP is added to the staff? The result is determined by many forces that are difficult to assess or predict. The first is the basic capability of the PA or NP, which includes training, experience, and personal characteristics, such as aptitude and drive. Next are the limitations imposed by the state medical board or the employer, designating that certain tasks will be the prerogative of the physician. Other variables external to the individual provider enhance or constrain the provider's basic efficiency. In part, the number of medical office visits handled by a provider during an hour or a day at an acceptable level of quality is determined by the range of types of presenting morbidities, the length of waiting room queue, the preferred practice style, the frequency and depth of physician supervision and, particularly if required supervisory intervention is frequent, the availability of the supervisor when needed. Other intrapractice variables can affect productivity:

- the size of the practice

- the length of the clinic day and number of call-back visits
- the type of visits, such as routine physical exams or acute illnesses
- the size and age of the local population
- the distribution of demographic characteristics, such as age, gender, and income
- the level of insurance coverage
- the supply of services by other local practices
- and general economic conditions.[16]

In the end, to properly evaluate the productivity of PAs and NPs, as many of the independent and dependent variables as possible should be incorporated. But even if they could all be identified, the influence of each variable on productivity would be difficult to evaluate with precision. With that caveat, it remains important that some estimate of productivity be ventured, whenever possible, to provide a reference point for planners, administrators, and employers seeking more efficient combinations of health care workers.

Table 2 presents the number of patients seen by appointment as medical office visits by various departments within KPNW in 1992. Though somewhat limited, these statistics provide a rough estimate of patient encounters on an hourly and daily rate.

In the departments of internal medicine and family practice, the PA and NP are on the same daily office schedule, and most patients are not triaged. Most medical office visits are scheduled every 15 minutes, with a maximum number of 25 visits in an eight-hour day for the primary care departments. If every available slot were filled, this schedule would exceed 4,000 medical office visits for primary care providers. In reality, each provider's schedule constantly erodes due to various factors. Inpatient service accounts for a large portion of this erosion, and if extended hours are worked, compensatory time off decreases annual medical office visit productivity. The employee benefit package allows six weeks off for physicians and two to five weeks off for PAs and NPs (see Compensation section). Sick leave, administrative time, sabbaticals, research, and other leaves of absence are additional contributing factors. Finally, the one-patient-every-15-minutes schedule varies depending on a number of factors, such as lengthier visits for procedures and physical examinations. Patients who do not keep their appointments may benefit the organization in reducing resource use but are included in calculating productivity.

Table 2
Outpatient Productivity
(end of year 12/31/92)

Department		FTE	Pt. Hours	Pt/Hr	Average Pt/Day	Appts Seen
Int Med	MD	100.00	243,780	2.39	17.4	200,583
	PA	13.0	13,697	2.61	19.0	21,428
	NP	15.5	15,551	2.26	17.0	20,382
Fam Prac	MD	59.2	72,785	3.10	22.5	115,342
	PA	18.4	26,915	2.97	21.5	39,220
	NP	1.6				
Pediatrics	MD	42.2	43,044	3.14	16.5	65,733
	PA	3.9	4,862	3.07	22.3	7,078
	NP	3.8	5,526	2.49	18.7	7,348
Ortho	MD	20.7	15,955	2.28	16.5	35,902
	PA	6.8	8,622	1.83	14.3	15,322
	DPM	5.4	6,771	2.04	14.8	13,426
OB/Gyn	MD	38.3	26,789	2.67	19.4	68,431
	CNM	6.4	4,021	2.48	16.1	9,608
	NP	12.4	15,551	2.26	17.0	32,074
Ophth	MD	8.9	10,780	3.30	23.9	31,522
	PA	1.0	1,523	2.91	21.1	1,320

Source: Kaiser Permanente, Northwest Region, Department of Medical Economics.

The result is a schedule of fewer than four patients per hour and fewer than 25 per day.

Annual medical office visits per type of provider (in FTE rates) are displayed in Table 2 but must be interpreted with caution, since the FTE rate is the amount of time providers worked, not necessarily the amount of time they saw scheduled patients. Patients seen in the emergency rooms, urgency care clinics, and special clinics are usually not attributed to any single provider.

When KPNW first examined productivity (patients seen per day) in the 1970s and its numbers revealed that PAs were as productive as physicians, the charge was levied that PAs were "skimming," or shifting easy-to manage patients to their schedule. If these charges were true, then physicians were seeing a disproportionate number of more complex cases. KPNW undertook a study to examine presenting morbidities managed by type of provider using a random 5 percent sample of all visits for one year. The results revealed that the frequency of preventive services managed by NPs was twice as high as MDs, and NP prenatal services were three times as high.

At the time of the study, most NPs were providing routine physical exams as part of the health appraisal program. PAs and MDs tended to see similar patients. They encountered a similar rate of acute viral and bacterial infections, although PAs tended to see proportionally more non-malignant chronic diseases (e.g., hypertension and diabetes). Both the PA and MD cohort saw an equal proportion of trauma and acute problems. The conditions most likely to be followed by the physician were systemic illnesses and episodes that included hospitalization (e.g., myocardial infarction, cerebral vascular accident). From these data, it appears that while there is some division of labor between PAs and MDs for about 10 percent of medical office visits in primary care, the remaining conditions are equally distributed; thus, skimming was not occurring.[17]

Prescribing

Very little empirical prescribing data are available about PAs or NPs, except some market surveys and a few limited research studies. Within KPNW, virtually all PAs and NPs have some prescription privileges. One study conducted in the late 1970s compared KPNW PAs and physicians for four acute illnesses. There was no statistical difference between prescribing rates and treatments by type of provider. There was, however, a slightly favorable safety outcome for PA prescribers when antibiotics were dispensed and adverse drug reactions were examined.[18]

To better understand PA and NP prescription rates and how they compare to physicians' in the same departments, a review of the KPNW computerized database of outpatient prescriptions was examined (Table 3). During August, September, and October 1992, a total of 454,395 prescriptions was attributed to four types of clinicians in four departments. These data suggest that PAs and NPs are responsible for at least 15 percent of all medication in primary care (adult and pediatrics), while staffing primary care at approximately 20 percent FTE. Orthopedic PAs represent one-fifth of the department

Table 3
Prescription Frequency (and Count) by Type of Provider
August, September, October 1992

Specialty	MD	DPM	PA	NP
IM	88.95% (213,481)	N/A	4.74% (11,370)	6.31%(15,146)
Ortho	70.52 (4,385)	15.13% (941)	14.35 (892)	N/A
Peds	85.92 (27,850)	N/A	8.10 (2,625)	5.98 (1,939)
FP	77.93 (136,980)	N/A	17.31 (30,428)	4.76 (8,358)
Total	84.22%	.20%	9.97%	5.59%

Source: Kaiser Permanente, Northwest Region, Department of Pharmacy Administration.

professionals (orthopedists, PAs, and podiatrists) and account for approximately one-sixth of the orthopedic prescriptions. Further investigation is needed to determine whether this discrepancy represents different morbidities seen by each type of provider, more conservative prescribing on the part of non-physician clinicians, or different prescribing rates per type of provider. However, KPNW pharmacists report that PAs and NPs write legibly, prescribe appropriately, and do so "more conservatively" when prescribing controlled substances, compared with physicians in the same department.

Member Satisfaction

Table 4 presents the results of a 57-item questionnaire sent to a random group of members within one week after their medical office visit. Samples were drawn from the automated appointment system, selected from all types of visits, all 17 medical offices, and all types of providers. This is a continuous rolling sample, and with special techniques to improve return, the response rate hovers around 70 percent. This approach has created a well-characterized reference population with good patient recall and motivation to respond.[19] This survey was examined from January 1991 through June 1992.

Four survey questions specifically concern satisfaction with care by the provider of last visit. A five-point scale allows respondents to choose among two levels of satisfaction, two levels of dissatisfaction, and indifference. When members were asked how satisfied they were with their latest encounter, adult practice PAs and NPs compared within one to two percentage points or physicians (between 88 per-

Table 4
Membership Satisfaction
Jan. 1991 - Jul. 1992

	IM		FP		PEDS	
	MD	**PA/NP**	**MD**	**PA**	**MD**	**PA/NP**
"How satisfied are you with the amount of time the provider spent with you?"						
Satisfied	91.3%	90.5%	89.1%	87.9%	88.7%	86.5%
Dissatisfied	2.9	4.1	3.7	4.3	4.85	5.4
"How satisfied are you with the amount of personal interest shown by the provider?"						
Satisfied	91.6	89.2	87.7	87.9	88.6	81.1
Dissatisfied	2.9	4.1	3.7	4.3	5.4	3.4
"How satisfied are you with the provider's technical competence, skill and ability?"						
Satisfied	93.6	89.7	89.9	86.7	92.1	81.9
Dissatisfied	1.7	1.8	2.2	4.3	2.3	4.2
"Overall, how satisfied are you with this visit?"						
Satisfied	90.3	87.9	86.9	86.7	88.6	78.4
Dissatisfied	4.1	5.7	4.8	5.5	5.4	8.1

Source: Marks S, Schmoldt R. *Kaiser Permanente Center for Health Research. Current Membership Study: 1992, Annual Report #27.* Portland, Ore: Kaiser Permanente; 1992.

cent and 90 percent favorable). The technical skill of PAs and NPs rated within three to four percentage points of MDs. As for overall satisfaction, members regard adult medicine PAs and NPs nearly the same as physicians. Pediatricians are viewed approximately 10 percent more favorably than pediatric PAs and NPs for reasons not clear at this time.

Compensation

One of the shortcomings of economic models that have examined PA, NP, and MD configurations is that they do not usually include benefits, which can be substantial if they involve housing, transportation, education, bonuses, and other incentives available to military and some rural practices. In this examination, the term "compensation" includes salary, benefits, and the monetary exchange an employer forgoes to retain an employee. Within KPNW, PAs and NPs are on parity for salary and benefits, regardless of responsibilities or job

Table 5

Benefit Package for KPNW PAs and NPs

Medical/Dental: Comprehensive coverage for the employee and eligible dependents.

Major Medical: Separate enrollment in a major medical plan for the employee and dependents. This plan covers medical expenses not covered by KP, including chiropractic and acupuncture.

Short term disability: Sick leave hours are accrued monthly, up to 96 hours per year.

Long term disability: 50 percent of salary for disabilities beyond 6 months.

Basic Life Insurance: Group life insurance based on age.

Optional Life Insurance: Additional discounted group life insurance is available.

Dependent Life Insurance: Coverage for spouse and dependent children is optional.

Salaried Retirement Plan: Employer contributes to a trust on behalf of the employee. Benefit at retirement is calculated based on a final average compensation and years of service.

Supplemental Savings and Retirement Plan: Employer contributes an amount equal to 5 percent of the employee's compensation when the employee contributes 2 percent to 5 percent of compensation. Employee is allowed to direct both employers and own contributions to one of six types of investment strategies.

Holidays: Nine paid holidays each year.

Vacation: Two to five weeks of paid vacation each year depending on length of employment.

Continuing Medical Education: One week of paid educational leave and $600 stipend annually.

Social Security: Mandatory matching, dollar for dollar, towards social security program.

Other Benefits: Employee Assistance Program (EAP), Dependent Care Reimbursement (DCRP), Tuition Reimbursement (up to $600 annually), Continuing Education, Worker's Compensation, Unemployment Insurance, Employee Health, Credit Union, and U.S. Saving Bond Payroll Savings Plan. These combined "other" benefits are estimated at $1,068 per annum and are available to all KP employees.

Source: Kaiser Permanente (Northwest) Department of Human Resources.

description. Physician earnings are based on a scale that depends on training, board certification, and years of experience. For PAs and NPs, salary is determined by years of experience; there are eight pay scales. Average PA earnings for 1992 are $49,500 nationally and $55,500 in the western United States.[20] Little is known about the average or range of salaries for NPs, but they are presumed to be comparable to those of PAs. The composition of benefits or perquisites at KPNW for PAs and NPs is listed in Table 5.

The value of KPNW paid benefits is approximately 36 percent of total KPNW compensation. Medical malpractice insurance has not been factored in but is another important item to calculate. The five-year average turnover is 11 percent for NPs and 5 percent for PAs. Industry and national statistics on benefits and retention are unavailable for either profession for comparison purposes.

Table 6 compares salaries. Physicians have a different salary scale and structure from health plan employees. Because the physician group is a for-profit corporation that contracts with the health plan, end-of-year revenues may be positive, and physicians can expect a bonus. The bonus for senior physicians (stockholders) varies annually; the $5,000 bonus listed for 1992 is above average. Conversely, in times of shortfall, physicians may have to accept an unpaid furlough for a few days.

Administration and Supervision

Supervision is that area of management that has wide interpretation depending on the state or federal department that regulates PAs or NPs. In Oregon, NPs may practice independently under the Nursing

Table 6
Primary Care Provider Compensation 1992

Type	Salary Range	Approximate % Benefits	Bonus*	Average+
Internist	$73,000-127,500	25	$5,000	$123,400
Family Practitioner	72,000-115,400	25	5,000	115,400
Pediatric	72,000-118,000	25	5,000	122,800
PA/NP	44,000-52,000	36	—	60,800

*Bonuses for physicians vary between $0 and $10,000 each year.
+Physician data include estimated call-back and in-house time, estimated benefits, and budgeted incentive compensation payment.

Source: *Northwest Permanente, PC.*

Act, but PAs must be employed by a supervising physician (in theory, the physician who provides direction and regular review). For PAs employed by the KPNW health plan, a supervising physician is assigned and agents are designated to act as supervising physician when the first physician is absent. For the most part, supervision is the relationship worked out between the PA and the MD assigned to him or her for that day. For policy convenience and quality of care, NPs are supervised in the same manner as PAs.

The administration of PAs and NPs varies widely among Kaiser Permanente regions. In some regions, they are employees of the physician group; in others, such as KPNW, they are health plan employees administered by the physician group. Six disciplines of non-physician providers are also loosely organized into an arrangement termed the Allied Health Council. This body, made up of representatives from NPs, PAs, nurse anesthetists, mental health, alcohol and chemical dependency counselors, and optometrist ranks, meets monthly to gather information about the organization and to disseminate it to constituents. The Allied Health Council also recognizes peers for contributions to their profession as well as to the organization.

Another form of administration within KPNW is the Coordinator of Allied Health Affairs, who serves as a manager for both the health plan and physician group. Tasks vary according to circumstances, but one role is to represent the non-physician provider's view during policy development.

Conclusion

KPNW is a non-profit, group-model health maintenance organization that makes use of a high diversity of health care providers and has developed mechanisms to ensure their roles in the organization. PAs and NPs are integrated into primary care practice arrangements (modules) that depend heavily on collaboration of providers. From the view of members, PAs and NPs appear to be delivering services as satisfactorily as physicians. From the view of administrators, they seem to be as productive as physicians, to prescribe similarly to physicians, and to be economically viable alternatives to physicians. Yet how do we establish the value of PA and NP services?

Certainly one critical aspect of cost containment for physician services is determination of access and quality of care. Thus, the value of PAs or NPs in terms of economic rewards ought to be derived from their contributions to access, quality, efficiency, equity, and ultimately, health status of patient clients.[21] Whether this is being accomplished at KPNW with more than 265 non-physician providers remains to be investigated.

The use of PAs and NPs in many KPNW departments is at a higher ratio to physicians than has been reported in the literature and at a level of productivity that compares to or exceeds physician rates in some instances. From a workload standpoint, it appears that adult medicine physicians, PAs, and NPs at KPNW see a similar number of patients on an hourly, daily, and annual basis, and the types of patients they see in adult ambulatory settings are probably similar as well. In this regard, PAs and NPs appear to substitute for, rather than complement, physicians. From an economic standpoint, they are employed at roughly 50 percent of physician costs (including salary and benefits). However, rapidly rising wages reflect that the market for PA and NP services is responding to shortages of health manpower, and this situation is expected to continue. The value to society may even be higher when one considers the total cost and duration of training (two years at $17,500 for a PA, versus eight years at $80,000 for a physician in 1992 dollars).

This examination of one organization raises many questions that require a more detailed understanding of specific activities and the allocation of time to each PA, NP, and physician. For instance, do PAs or NPs negate any of their cost-effectiveness in the way they approach similar conditions? Do they order more laboratory tests and procedures per episode of illness or prescribe more expensive medications than physicians for the same diagnosis and within the same age group? Do physicians use telephone encounters differently than do PAs or NPs? Do PAs' and NPs' patients tend to return more often than physicians' patients? Which provider is more likely to refer certain conditions for consultation? Another factor that was not addressed in this paper is the cost implication of the requirement for physician consultation and supervision in patient care rendered by the PA or NP.

Finally, the utilization of PAs and NPs is often limited on grounds generally unrelated to issues of quality. In many states, medical licensing boards retain control over the introduction and use of such personnel. To produce physician-type services at minimum cost, it is necessary to be able to legally employ the desired quantity of health manpower and to be able to delegate the tasks to them that they are trained to perform. Any restrictions limiting the use of such persons should be removed while at the same time holding the institution, *and not the physician*, responsible for maintaining quality. For example, the HMO contracts with members, so it seems reasonable that the HMO should provide the assurance that quality is not being compromised.

Perhaps the enhanced monitoring systems being developed in many institutions that depend on improved and expanded documentation in the medical record could be used to monitor physician and non-physician practitioners equally. In the end, improving the medical record for quick retrieval and complying with the requirements of an enhanced system will allow greater analysis of workloads in ways as yet unrealized. If the final analysis reveals that medical outcomes for most primary care conditions are similar when treated by an MD, a PA, or an NP, then this may well be the stimulus for changing the ratio of medical school enrollments to PA and NP program enrollments that has been advocated by the underwriter of this conference.[22]

References

1. Lairson P, Record JC, James JC. Physician assistants at Kaiser: distinctive patterns of practice. *Inquiry.* 1974;11:207-219.

2. Record JC, Cohen HR. The introduction of midwifery in a prepaid group practice. *Am J Pub Health.* 1972;62:354-360.

3. Hooker RS. Medical care utilization: MD-PA/NP comparisons in an HMO. In: Zarbock SF, Harbert K, eds. *Physician Assistants: Present and Future Models of Utilization.* Philadelphia, PA: Praeger; 1986.

4. Smith KR, Miller M, Golladay FL. An analysis of the optimal use of inputs in production of medical services. *J Human Resources.* 1972;7:208-224. Golliday FL, Miller M, Smith KR. Allied health manpower strategies: estimates of the potential gains from efficient task delegation. *Medical Care.* 1973;11:457-469.

5. Reinhardt UE. A production function for physician services. *Review Economics and Statistics.* 1972;February:63.

6. Reinhardt UE. *Physician Productivity and the Demand for Health Manpower.* Cambridge, MA: Ballinger; 1975.

7. Scheffler RM. The employment, utilization, and earnings of physician extenders. *Soc Sci Med.* 1977;11:785-791.

8. Record JC, O'Bannon JE, Mullooly JP. *Cost Effectiveness of Physician's Assistants in a Large HMO: Phase I of a Two-Phase Study.* Springfield, Va: National Technical Information Service. NO HRA-090098, 1978.

9. Page RR. *The Military Physician's Assistant.* Preliminary report for Health Studies Task Force, Office of the Assistant Secretary of Defense for Health and Environment. Washington, DC: Department of Defense; 1975.

10. Hooker RS. Medical care utilization: MD-PA/NP comparisons in an HMO. In: Zarbock SF, Harbert K, eds. *Physician Assistants: Present and Future Models of Utilization.* Philadelphia, PA: Praeger; 1986.

11. Reinhardt UE. A production function for physician services. *Review Economics and Statistics.* 1972;February:63. Scheffler RM. The employment, utilization, and earnings of physician extenders. *Soc Sci Med.* 1977;11:785-791.

12. A note of caution is introduced here to avoid the temptation to use a physician-ratio calculation and then to compare with other organizations. All organizations, even within different KP regions, use physician services differently. Some HMOs refer certain conditions out to the community for capitated services, such as cardiac arterial bypass graft surgery. Other regions may not even own a hospital; this situation affects staffing ratios considerably. Within each KP region, the number and roles of non-physician providers differ markedly, depending on policy or state laws. Even if one wanted to compare manpower delivery for primary care services, adjustments would need to be made for the age distribution and socioeconomic status of the membership, the amount of administrative responsibility physicians have and even the age of the physician group.

13. Johnson RE, Freeborn DK, McCally M. Delegation of office visits in primary care to PAs and NPs: the physicians' view. *Physician Assistant.* 1985;January:159-169.

14. Hooker RS. Employment specialization in the PA profession: the educational process, market forces, and complex fields that influence the trend to specialize. *J Am Acad Physician Assistants.* 1992;5:695-703.

15. Record JC. *Staffing Primary Care in 1990: Physician Replacement and Cost Savings.* New York, NY: Springer Publishing Company; 1981.

16. Record JC, Hurtado AV, O'Bannon JE. Quality of PA performance at a health maintenance organization. In: Bliss AA, Cohen ED, eds. *The New Health Professionals: Nurse Practitioners and Physician's Assistants.* Germantown, Md: Aspen Systems Corporation; 1977.

17. Hooker RS. Medical care utilization: MD-PA/NP comparisons in an HMO. In: Zarbock SF, Harbert K, eds. *Physician Assistants: Present and Future Models of Utilization.* Philadelphia, PA: Praeger; 1986.

18. Record JC, Hurtado AV, O'Bannon JE. Quality of PA performance at a health maintenance organization. In: Bliss AA, Cohen ED, eds. *The New Health Professionals: Nurse Practitioners and Physician's Assistants.* Germantown, Md: Aspen Systems Corporation; 1977.

19. Marks S, Schmoldt R. Kaiser Permanente Center for Health Research. *Current Membership Study: 1992, Annual Report #27.* Portland, Ore: Kaiser Permanente; 1992.

20. Willis J. 1992 PA census data: settings and salaries. *Am Acad Physician Assistants News.* November, 1992.

21. Hornbrook MC. Economic models of nursing practice: substitution, competition, and co-management. In: Lindman C. *Work and Society: Implications for Professional Nursing.* Washington, DC: American Association of Colleges of Nursing; 1988:55-110.

22. Miekel TR, Jr. President's Statement. *Josiah Macy, Jr. Foundation Annual Report, 1992.* New York, NY; 1993.

6

Meeting the Needs of the Underserved: The Roles of Physician Assistants and Nurse Practitioners

Virginia Fowkes

ENSURING ACCESS TO HEALTH SERVICES IS A MAJOR objective of health policy in the United States. Although national efforts since the 1960s have enhanced the general availability of medical care, several notable segments of the population continue to face considerable barriers to access. These segments include the uninsured, the poor living in urban and rural areas, and some ethnic minorities. Approximately 10 to 15 percent of the U.S. population is without access to appropriate health care, and substantial differences in health status are still related to ethnicity.[1] In addition to financial and geographic barriers experienced by other segments of the population, minority populations experience cultural and attitudinal barriers to health care.

The physician assistant (PA) and nurse practitioner (NP) professions were developed for two main reasons: to expand the availability of primary care services and to improve access to these services for medically underserved populations. There are approximately 24,000 PAs. Data regarding practice specialty are available for about 80 percent of them. More than half (56 percent) are practicing in primary care, fifteen percent are in towns of less than 10,000 residents, and 31 percent are in communities of less than 50,000 population.[2] These data are derived from member surveys by the American Academy of Physician Assistants (AAPA), representing approximately half of all physician assistants.

Several PA programs with track records of deploying graduates in primary care and underserved sites have noted that many of their graduates (particularly ethnic minority graduates) are not AAPA members. Programs have also noted discrepancies between their own data and the national database. The consequent possibility of selection bias suggests that PA involvement in primary care or rural communities may be even higher than the data indicate.

Most PAs (55 percent) have baccalaureate or higher degrees at the time of program admission, and many, particularly in the Medex-type programs, have substantial clinical backgrounds, averaging 52 months of health care experience at program entry. More than half of enrolled PA students are over 27 years of age, and the proportion of students over 29 has increased over the past nine years. The majority (62 percent) of the approximately 3,400 current PA students are women, and about 20 percent are ethnic minorities.[3] A recent survey of California graduates found that 30 percent were ethnic minorities.[4]

NPs are the most numerous and diverse group of midlevel providers. NP specialties include family, pediatrics, adult, geriatrics, women's health, psychiatry and mental health, obstetrics and gynecology, midwifery, and other areas. Data from the 1988 national sample of registered nurses identified a population of 56,043 with NP training, of whom 20,838 were in current practice in a variety of specialties.[5] Comparisons between those practicing in metropolitan counties (population greater than 50,000) and non-metropolitan counties (population less than 50,000) yielded the following findings:

- The distribution of NPs was heavily skewed in favor of metropolitan counties (91 percent).
- In both settings, the majority (98 percent) were female, and the mean age was 42.
- More non-metropolitan NPs (72 percent) were married than metropolitan NPs (63 percent).
- More metropolitan NPs (46 percent) had baccalaureate and higher degrees than did non-metropolitan NPs (31 percent). And, predictably, more non-metropolitan NPs had diplomas (46 percent) and associate degrees (23 percent) than metropolitan NPs (39 percent and 15 percent, respectively).
- NPs in metropolitan areas averaged annual salaries of $3,400

greater than non-metropolitan NPs.

- While NPs in metropolitan areas were evenly distributed among four primary care specialties (family, women's health, adult, and pediatric care), the major proportion of non-metropolitan NPs (47 percent) were family NPs.[6]

A 1990 national survey by the American Academy of Nurse Practitioners found that, compared to graduates of master's-level preparation, NPs prepared in certificate programs were more likely to practice full time and to work in rural areas and small towns. Of NPs in small communities, 66 percent were certificate-prepared. Full-time practice was reported by only 56 percent of master's-prepared NPs compared to 73 percent of NPs with diplomas or associate degrees and 65 percent of those from baccalaureate programs.[7]

Another study comparing 112 master's- and non-master's-prepared pediatric nurse practitioner graduates yielded similar findings: The non-master's group was more likely to be employed in primary health care and to practice in rural areas.[8] Several studies have found no differences in clinical or board examination performances between NP graduates of certificate or master's programs.[9]

In recent years, while overall minority enrollment has declined, certificate programs have experienced a steady rise in minority enrollment and graduation.[10]

No reliable summary information about the clinical or academic backgrounds of NP students appears to be available. A recent survey of 147 NP programs noted that ethnic minority students (blacks, Hispanics, Asians, and Native Americans) represented 15 percent of NP students in 1990. The highest concentrations were in California, New York, Florida and Massachusetts — states with large numbers of minority populations.[11] A survey of registered nurses, the pool from which NP students are drawn, found that about 8 percent were members of minority groups.[12] It is not known whether those increases can be generalized to NP students.

Similarities and Differences between PAs and NPs

The PA and NP professions were developed for similar purposes. Many studies have documented their impact, the quality of care they provide, the cost effectiveness of this care, and patient satisfaction with services from each group. Evaluation of care provided by PAs and NPs suggests that, within their areas of competence, they provide care that is equivalent in quality to that of physicians, with patient support and communication functions perhaps superior to that of many physicians.[13]

Many settings employ both PAs and NPs, with similar job descriptions and mechanisms for physician collaboration and supervision. Thus, the *functions* of PAs and NPs within the same specialty and in the same setting are similar. Other similarities appear in some programs' goals and curricula, particularly within the same specialty (e.g., management of patients with chronic disease or skills in taking a patient history or performing a physical examination). These commonalities are particularly evident among programs focused on training for underserved areas.[14]

The differences between PAs and NPs are more confusing, involving diverse qualifications as well as institutional, legal, professional, and political factors. For example, NPs are licensed, registered nurses, whereas PAs enter training from a variety of backgrounds. Most PA programs were established by schools of medicine, and most training programs have been established within, or with strong attachments to, medical schools. Nationally, most provide baccalaureate degrees which give the student two years of general education and two years of clinical training. Clinical training is similar to that of medical students, with rotating clerkships and didactic courses. Programs in the Western states, however, have generally followed the Medex model of training, recruiting trainees with prior academic and clinical work and providing most clinical training by preceptorships in community office or clinic settings. Often in these programs there is a pre-selection student-preceptor commitment.[15]

Educational preparation for NPs, in contrast, was established largely by schools of nursing. While a few certificate programs remain, the majority of NP education occurs at the master's level, with NP students developing skills in advanced nursing practice.

PA and NP programs differ among themselves in specialty focus, though most focus on primary care. Other PA program types include emergency medicine, women's health, neonatal, and surgery. NP program specialties include family, adult, obstetrics and gynecology, midwifery, pediatrics, geriatrics, mental health, and others.

Each discipline has its own national educational organization, accrediting body, and certification procedures. The Association of Physician Assistant Programs is the organization of PA educational programs. The Committee on Allied Health Education and Accreditation of the American Medical Association is the agency responsible for accrediting PA programs. The National Commission on the Certification of Physician Assistants administers the national board examinations in primary care and other specialties which are accepted by most states as requisite for individual PA licensure.

For NPs, the National Organization of Nurse Practitioner Faculties is the association of NP educators. The National League for Nursing is responsible for accreditation of nursing programs. The American Nurses Credentialing Center sponsors examinations in several specialties for individual NP national certification. In addition, some specialties have their own national certification examinations. However, states vary considerably in licensure requirements for NP practice. California, for example, does not require national certification for NP practice.

There are differences in licensure requirements, reimbursement, and authorized activities. While these factors differ substantially from state to state, generally PAs practice under some provision of the states' Medical Practice Acts and under the direct supervision of physicians. NPs, on the other hand, practice under nursing licensure and provisions made in Nurse Practice Acts. Provisions are made for collaborative practice where the functions of nursing and medical practice overlap.

Each discipline has its own professional organization. For PAs, the most widely recognized is the American Academy of Physician Assistants and for NPs, a number of specialty professional organizations are joined under an umbrella organization, the National Alliance of Nurse Practitioners.

Finally, there are political differences. These have been generated by the unfortunate beginnings in antagonism and conflict between organized medicine and nursing, as well as by differences in the educational assumptions of the two types of training programs. Political differences are accentuated locally when there is competition for employment sites or controversy in state legislatures about privileges for practice, reimbursement, or prescribing.[16]

PA/NP Practice with the Underserved
PAs and NPs have provided increased access to health services in a wide variety of geographic and practice settings, both in rural and

inner-city areas, and in health programs for the poor, minorities and people without health insurance. They have augmented services in settings where physicians are less likely to practice, such as community and migrant health centers (CMHCs), public institutions, school-based clinics, long-term-care facilities and nursing homes, correctional institutions, and industrial health clinics. These diverse settings, roles, and populations are referred to simply as "underserved."

More than half of the graduates of PA training programs since 1985 have gone into primary care practice.[17] In 1988, 15 percent of practicing NPs worked in non-metropolitan counties.[18]

PAs and NPs make a significant contribution to rural health care provided by CMHCs. One recent study found that CMHCs average 2.2 full-time equivalent, non-physician primary care providers per site and hope to hire 315 NPs and 218 PAs over the next three years.[19] In studying factors related to retaining PAs and NPs for employment in CMHCs, this study found links to community, spouse employment and satisfaction, availability of continuing education, positive work environment, and the presence of student training programs to be important. Eighty percent of McKinney Act Clinics providing primary care to the homeless employ NPs.[20] A recent study showed that NPs can provide care to persons with AIDS that is of the same caliber as care provided by MDs, but at a lower cost.[21]

Many studies have found that health professionals from the same cultural background are better able to communicate with their patients and have a positive influence on health outcomes.[22] Minority PAs have been reported to be more likely than their non-minority peers to work in public institutions and clinics and in primary care specialties. They also have been reported to see a greater percentage of patients who are non-white and from low-income families.[23] Black PAs were disproportionately found serving in federal, state, city and private hospitals, community clinics, nursing homes, military hospitals, clinics, and federal and city prisons.[24]

A recent study of 641 PAs in California revealed 14 percent working in community clinics and 13 percent in county systems. This study also characterized features about PA practice with underserved populations. Most PAs reported using a language other than English with their patients — usually Spanish — and notably 34 percent of the total reported speaking Spanish with fluency. PA respondents also estimated proportions of their most recent week of regular practice spent with designated groups; proportions exceeding 15 percent were interpreted to be substantial. Thirty-two percent of PAs reported substantial involvement with patients not fluent in English, 61 percent reported substantial parts of their practice with ethnic minorities, 46 percent with patients receiving Medicaid, and 22 percent with patients whose care was unreimbursed.[25]

Educational Strategies for Deployment to Underserved Areas

For the Health Resources and Services Administration, my colleagues Gamel, Wilson, Garcia and I recently completed a study of 51 PA, NP, and certified nurse midwife (CNM) programs to identify and evaluate strategies to prepare and deploy trainees for work in underserved areas.[26] This study included 20 PA, 22 NP, seven CNM, and two combined PA/NP programs known to have an orientation toward underserved areas. A national advisory panel of seven academic and professional leaders from each of the three disciplines assisted in study design and interpretation of results. Using protocols keyed to specific study questions, we reviewed program documents, conducted 170 interviews, and visited nine programs selected for their diversity. Assessments included student demographic data, faculty backgrounds, program structure, recruitment and retention strategies, curriculum development, educational process and deployment mechanisms. In addition, we requested graduate practice data.

Programs were defined as successful if more than 60 percent of graduates were in primary care practices and a substantial number were in underserved settings (e.g., 25 percent in health professional shortage areas, more than 25 percent in towns of less than 10,000 or more than 60 percent in different types of underserved areas). The most successful programs were those having comprehensive strategies related to the goal of deploying graduates to work with underserved populations that were interwoven throughout their selection and educational processes, programs that had adapted their structure and function to fit their chosen missions. There were proportionally more PA programs with comprehensive strategies and evidence of successful outcomes than NP programs (41 percent versus 21 percent).

Part of the problem in evaluating success was the lack of data about graduate practice. More than one-third (36 percent) of PA programs and more than one-half (58 percent) of NP programs did not submit these data, usually because they had none.

Programs' Structural Characteristics
Having a formally stated program mission proved a strong prediction of effective focus on the underserved. Almost three-fourths of programs with clear mission statements about preparing students for practice in underserved areas also conducted most of their students' training in underserved sites and had outcome data on graduate practice. Indeed, having a mission statement was significantly associated with having graduate practice data (p<.01).

Nearly half of the programs studied were either located in or had a major component in an underserved area or in an institution caring for large indigent populations. Such a location can assist in recruiting students from the target area, locating clinical training sites there, and deploying graduates. Programs that are not strategically located can gain similar advantages by locating some recruiting and training activities in target underserved areas. However, the simple fact of location in an underserved area without other targeting strategies did not appear to lead to successful placement of graduates in the area. Similarly, programs with comprehensive strategies for deploying graduates to underserved areas were able to do so without being located in such an area.

The Medex program model, prevalent in PA and some NP training in the Western United States, appears to have major advantages for placing graduates in underserved areas. In fact, most of the study programs found to be successful were of the Medex type (56 percent of successful PA and 60 percent of successful NP programs). Some of these programs did not originate as PA Medex programs. However, they typically featured a commitment to underserved areas or settings and a practice of selecting preceptors and students together before admission (with an expectation of employment upon graduation). Frequently, students receive almost all clinical training in the community-based preceptorship, usually in or near the student's home community. Students matriculate with considerable academic and clinical experience. With an abundance of jobs for PAs and NPs, some programs have more recently found the student-preceptor selection match unnecessary.

Characteristics of program faculty influence all aspects of their programs. Faculty can provide both professional and ethnic role models for students. Programs in the study that lacked ethnic minority faculty noted that this factor hindered their efforts to recruit minority students. Additionally, programs with minority faculty were more likely than others to devote time to cross-cultural instruction and experiences.

Most respondents in the study agreed that rural and underserved areas need primary care practitioners having a broad range of skills and the ability to function independently. Many NP programs training students in pediatrics or women's health, for example, found that graduates practicing in underserved areas were returning for training in family practice.

Our study was limited by design to programs concerned with underserved areas and populations. In relation to the needs of the underserved, the numbers of practitioners being graduated from these programs (about 680 PAs and 500 NPs per year) are small. And, of course, not all of these graduates will choose to practice or to remain with the underserved.

Recruitment and Retention

Graduates who elect to practice with underserved populations appeared to be older and to have some prior experience with such populations. During site visits, more than three-fourths of students and graduates we interviewed indicated that personal or background characteristics they had brought to their training were the factors that led them to choose to practice in underserved areas.

Certain strategies were common among the programs successful in recruiting and retaining students oriented to the underserved. These included providing financial aid, having flexible admission requirements, offering part-time or extended programs, admitting student-preceptor pairs together (the Medex model), providing extra academic support for target students, offering outreach baccalaureate completion programs for rural nurses, having ethnic minority faculty members, and recruiting in underserved areas. Financial aid is particularly important in attracting students most likely to practice in underserved areas, since many of these students are older and have family and other financial obligations.

The conversion of certificate NP programs to graduate degree programs was a barrier to the recruiting of rural and ethnic minority nurses, many of whom have associate degrees. For example, the very successful NP program training rural nurses in North Dakota converted to a PA program because of this problem. Other admission requirements of graduate programs (minimum scores on standardized tests or undergraduate grade point averages) also hinder NP program involvement with target students, many of whom are educationally disadvantaged.

Education and Deployment
Programs in our study with missions to serve rural areas often had special courses, seminars, and case presentations devoted to needs of rural populations. Faculty in these programs were often from rural areas and had rural practice experience. All programs in the study conducted some clinical training in underserved areas. Almost half the PA programs in the study had required preceptorships in underserved sites, perhaps in response to the FY 1993 federal funding preference for four-week preceptorships in underserved areas. Students and graduates interviewed in this study stressed the importance of clinical training in underserved sites in preparing them for practice with underserved populations; however, the influence of such training on actual choices of practice location, particularly in the absence of other strategies, is unclear.

All programs in the study had PA, NP, or CNM role models, both as faculty members and preceptors. Many program faculty practiced with underserved populations and, particularly in CNM programs, some supervised students in their practices. In some instances, faculty trained medical students and residents as well, helping to prepare students for interdisciplinary team practice.

Rural and remote practice locations demand a wide variety of skills in health care practitioners who will need to be relatively independent. Conversion of many NP programs to the graduate level resulted in the reduction of the amount of clinical training offered to students, since new courses in nursing theory, research, and statistics are required. Thus, some NP programs may not provide sufficient clinical training for practice in underserved areas.

Issues and Problems

In the 1980s, growing recognition of the PA and NP professions expanded employment opportunities to a variety of specialties. Funding for CHCs and NHSC positions decreased substantially, and the

Graduate Medical Education National Advisory Committee (GEMENAC)'s predicting a surplus of physicians, discouraged further development of the professions and contributed to a decrease in the numbers choosing to work in these settings.

The 1990s present a different picture. Changes in reimbursement practices associated with health care reform and the trend toward managed care are likely to increase the demand for PA and NP services, but this demand will increase in specialty as well as in primary care sectors.

Historically, PAs have been called upon to function as house staff in teaching hospitals that have reduced the size of residency programs or in inner-city institutions losing the services of foreign medical graduates because of restrictions on their practices. As reimbursement mechanisms for graduate medical education change, accompanied by loss of residency positions in both medical and surgical subspecialties, medical centers are likely to recruit PAs to replace these positions and make up for the implicit loss of services. Educational programs for PAs, many of which are based within the labyrinth of university medical centers, will be asked to respond to new service needs. This potential diversion of PA resources away from primary care raises a question about the need to recognize and subsidize separately the training of two PA professional groups — the primary care specialists and the inpatient, hospital-based specialists.

NPs are less likely to experience such transitions, since advanced practice nursing already includes clinical specialists who function within subspecialty areas, such as coronary care, and are most often hospital-based.

Several issues interfere with successful recruitment, training, and deployment of PAs and NPs to underserved areas. A major one is cost. Programs most likely to deploy their graduates among the underserved use expensive strategies to produce that result, such as decentralization, outreach, and dispersal of students over a wide geographic area for clinical training. Students most likely to practice in underserved areas are least likely to be able to afford the costs of their training, particularly when, in addition to tuition or fees, the training requires them to give up their employment for a year or more. Without the financial support of the federal and state governments, many of the most successful programs would not survive.

Diversion of students from primary care to subspecialties is an increasing problem that is exacerbated by training in tertiary care institutions. The higher salaries offered by subspecialties are attractive to students who have incurred debts during their training. Some graduates address this problem by practicing half time in a private practice and half time in an underserved site. Primary care programs reinforce this emphasis by clarifying students' practice goals at the time of admission, analyzing the profiles of students who actually enter primary care practice and practice in underserved areas, providing more training in geographic target areas, and strengthening their program mission with classroom activities and faculty who model program goals.

With most NP programs now at the graduate level, increased academic requirements in this type of training hinder the recruiting of older rural and ethnic minority students most likely to practice with underserved populations. Lack of ethnic minority faculty and/or lack of sensitivity to cultural issues may compound the recruitment problem. Graduate programs struggling for institutional recognition may come to value their faculty's academic and research achievements more than cross-cultural and clinical experience with underserved populations, thus diminishing their ability to recruit appropriate faculty role models for their students.

The success of continued and increasing deployment and retention of PAs and NPs in underserved settings will ultimately be influenced by factors outside the trainees and their preparation. These factors include adequate reimbursement for their services, flexibility in state practice laws and regulations, and professional issues.

Available data suggest that just one-third of the NPs who have been trained to care for underserved patients are practicing.[27] Several factors may contribute to this attrition. First, the array of NP specialties may not fit the job market. Second, nurses can often make higher salaries by returning to previous roles in hospital nursing than by practicing in primary care. Third, both the PA and nursing literature identify considerable restrictions on their respective scopes of practice.

Lack of prescriptive authority and eligibility for reimbursement are frequent barriers to practice in rural and underserved areas. For example, the AAPA in 1990 noted that in states where PAs have prescribing privileges, 17.3 percent of practicing PAs were in rural areas; whereas in states where PAs do not have privileges, only 8 percent were in rural areas.[28]

Both the PA and NP professions are relatively young. They are allied with the older professions of medicine and nursing that have already made some mistakes. Here I wish to add a personal note. As one with a background in nursing, a career centered in medical education, and long involvement with community programs, I have been repeatedly impressed with the consequences of academic medicine and nursing pursuing professional interests at the expense of community service.

The training of practitioners for underserved areas requires flexibility in institutional practices. Many programs are struggling to continue their missions with formidable institutional barriers — barriers at the national level, due to accreditation requirements in nursing; barriers at the state level, due to restrictive practice laws; and local barriers, due to competition from other faculty who do not share an interest in primary care or with whom program directors must compete for resources.

For many years, academic medicine turned its back on primary care service needs. Medical schools valued the research interests of faculty and the training of subspecialists. Faculty and students interested in primary care were often viewed as second-class citizens. Only recently have political pressure and the rising costs of health care forced the schools to begin to address population service needs and the need for more primary care practitioners. PA programs, primarily created by medical schools, offer a small solution to the problem, but PA programs express concern about their graduates following in the footsteps of role models in medical centers and being lured away from primary care to subspecialty practice.

Academic nursing, although more recent in its evolution, may be making some of the same mistakes made by academic medicine. The National League of Nursing (NLN) and the American Nurses Association (ANA) have set academic and professional standards that have compromised programs with missions highly focused on underserved populations, such as the North Dakota program mentioned previously. As of 1992, NPs are required to have a master's in nursing as part of, or in addition to, their NP training to be eligible to take the ANA national certifying examinations. NPs without an M.S.N. who are trained in certificate programs are not eligible to take this examination (which states are increasingly requiring for NP practice) despite evidence suggesting that certificate programs have a better track record than master's level programs in placing graduates in underserved sites.

The struggle for professionalism has been equated with higher degrees and has resulted in divisiveness in many areas of nursing education and practice. Some suggest that the higher the degree, the further away from the client the practitioner becomes. Faculty in schools of nursing with NP programs are preferred at the doctoral level. In many nursing schools, faculty are valued (as shown by requirements for tenure) first for their ability to do research, second for their skills as teachers, and third for their skills as clinicians. NPs who have doctoral degrees and are skilled clinicians are extremely scarce. Clinical teachers for most NPs in our study population were master's-prepared clinicians who have "lower status" in their schools or who are community-based and have clinical rather than tenured appointments in order to comply with university requirements. Some programs were developing community-based service models for teaching and research. Locating these efforts in underserved sites and expanding these models will likely improve deployment and retention of graduates in these sites.

Conclusion

The role of PAs and NPs in providing care to underserved populations has been well established. There is considerable information about who goes to underserved areas and about the educational strategies that work to get them there. NP programs are placing graduates in all sectors of primary care. However, the academic evolution of the NP role, while understandable, may have diminished its relevance to underserved populations. Programs shaped specifically to a mission targeting the underserved have been more successful. Both trainees and educational programs that are likely to continue the mission need increased support in the forms both of financial aid and training resources. Programs will require more government and institutional financing and the increased availability of underserved community sites for clinical training. Successful deployment of graduates will also require comprehensive educational strategies that narrow the gap between educational and service needs and a commitment from both PA and NP professions that balances professional interests with these service needs.

References

1. U.S. Department of Health and Human Services, Office of Inspector General. *State Regulation of Nonphysician Health Care Practitioners: Inspection Design*. Boston, Mass.: Office of Evaluation and Inspections; 1991.

2. American Academy of Physician Assistants. *General Census Data on Physician Assistants 1991*. Washington, D.C.: AAPA; 1991.

3. Oliver DR. *Eighth Annual Report on Physician Assistant Educational Programs in the United States, 1991-1992*. Iowa City, Iowa: Association of Physician Assistant Programs; 1992.

4. Fowkes VK, McKay D. A profile of California's physician assistants. *Western J of Med*. 1990;153:328-329.

5. Ahmed KA, Muus KJ. Comparison of metro and non-metro nurse practitioner characteristics. *Focus on Rural Health*. 1991;8:6-7.

6. Ahmed KA, Muus KJ. Comparison of metro and non-metro nurse practitioner characteristics. *Focus on Rural Health*. 1991;8:6-7.

7. Schnare S. *Entry into practice dilemmas: a review of research and health care environment impacts*. Unpublished manuscript, Harbor-UCLA Medical Center, Torrance, Calif.; 1991.

8. Cruikshank BM, Lakin JA. Professional and employment characteristics of NPs with master's and nonmaster's preparation. *Nurse Practitioner*. 1986;11:45-52.

9. Schnare S. *Entry into practice dilemmas: a review of research and health care environment impacts*. Unpublished manuscript, Harbor-UCLA Medical Center, Torrance, Calif.; 1991.

10. Schnare S. *Entry into practice dilemmas: a review of research and health care environment impacts*. Unpublished manuscript, Harbor-UCLA Medical Center, Torrance, Calif.; 1991.

11. Harper DC, Zimmer PA. Summary of NP educational program survey results. *NONPF Newsletter*. 1992;3.

12. Moses EB. *1988: The Registered Nurse Population*. Washington, DC: Bureau of Health Professions; 1990.

13. U.S. Congress, Office of Technology Assessment. *Nurse Practitioners, Physician Assistants, and Certified Nurse Midwives: A Policy Analysis*. Washington DC: US Government Printing Office; 1986. Publication OTA-HCS-37.

14. Fowkes VK, Mentink J. Nurses and physician assistants: issues and challenges. In: McCloskey J, Grace H, eds. *Current Issues in Nursing*, 4th ed. Hanover, Md: Mosby-Year Book Inc.; (in press).

15. Fowkes VK, Mentink J. Nurses and physician assistants: issues and challenges. In: McCloskey J, Grace H, eds. *Current Issues in Nursing*, 4th ed. Hanover, Md: Mosby-Year Book Inc.; (in press).

16. Fowkes VK, Mentink J. Nurses and physician assistants: issues and challenges. In: McCloskey J, Grace H, eds. *Current Issues in Nursing*, 4th ed. Hanover, Md: Mosby-Year Book Inc.; (in press).

17. Oliver DR. *Seventh Annual Report on Physician Assistant Educational Programs in the United States, 1990-91*. Iowa City, Iowa: Association of Physician Assistant Programs; 1991.

18. Moses EB. *1988: The Registered Nurse Population. Washington, DC: Bureau of Health Professions; 1990*.

19. Samuels ME, Shi L. *Report on the Survey of Community and Migrant Health Centers Regarding Utilization of Nurse Practitioners, Physicians Assistants, and Certified Nurse Midwives*. Columbia, SC: Department of Health Administration, School of Public Health, University of South Carolina; 1991.

20. Dobin BH, Gelberg L, Freeman HE. Patient care and professional staffing patterns in McKinney Act clinics providing primary care to the homeless. *JAMA*. 1992;267:698-701.

21. Scherer P. Comparing NP with MD care for people with AIDS. *Am J Nursing*. 1990;90:43.

22. Agency for Health Care Policy and Research. *Annotated Bibliography of AHCPR Research on Nonphysician Primary Care Providers 1969-1989*. Rockville, Md.: US Department of Health and Human Services; 1990.

23. U.S. Department of Health and Human Services, Office of Inspector General. *State Regulation of Nonphysician Health Care Practitioners: Inspection Design*. Boston, Mass.: Office of Evaluation and Inspections; 1991.

24. Schafft GE, Cawley JF. *The Physician Assistant in a Changing Health Care Environment*. Rockville, Md.: Aspen; 1987.

25. Fowkes VK, McKay D. A profile of California's physician assistants. *Western J of Med*. 1990;153:328-329.

26. Fowkes VK, Gamel N, Wilson S, Garcia R. *Assessment of Physician Assistant, Nurse Practitioner, and Nurse-Midwife Training on Meeting Health Care Needs of the Underserved*. Final report of HRSA contract no. 240-91-0050. Stanford, Calif.: 1993.

27. Ahmed KA, Muus KJ. Comparison of metro and non-metro nurse practitioner characteristics. *Focus on Rural Health.* 1991;8:6-7.

28. Willis JB. Prescriptive practice patterns of physician assistants. *J Am Acad Physician Assistants.* 1990;3:39-56.

7

Physician Assistant Education: A Review of Program Characteristics by Sponsoring Institution

Denis Oliver

THE PHYSICIAN ASSISTANT (PA) CONCEPT EMERGED IN the mid-1960s, in response to a widespread need for cost-effective, accessible primary health care in the United States.[1] Initially, the role PAs would play was unclear, as was the extent to which they would be incorporated into, and accepted by, various groups in the health care system, such as patients, physicians, nurses, and other allied health care professionals. Within a relatively short time, however, health manpower studies provided compelling evidence to support expectations that, given appropriate legal parameters in which to practice, PAs could provide high quality[2] and cost-effective[3] health care to a substantial proportion of patients without over-the-shoulder supervision by physicians.[4]

In the early stages of the profession, a variety of educational approaches evolved to prepare PAs for practice. At Duke University, in 1965, Eugene Stead established the first PA program in a major medical center.[5] The course of study consisted of seven months of basic and clinical science instruction, followed by 13 months of rotating clerkships, and culminated in a two-month preceptorship, typically in an office-based practice.

The Medex (medical extension) model of education, established at the University of Washington and the University of Utah in 1969, involved three months of intensive basic and clinical science instruction, followed by 12 to 15 months of a community-based preceptorship with a prospective employing physician.[6]

A specialty model, focusing on pediatrics, was developed at the University of Colorado Medical School in 1969.[7] The three-year curriculum followed a sequence of courses similar to the medical curriculum and enrolled individuals with a nursing credential and work experience in pediatrics.

In that same year, a PA program was established at a four-year liberal arts college, independent of a major medical center.[8] While the program enrolled principally high school graduates, the first two years of the curriculum were focused on liberal arts and general science courses, and the final two years involved the PA professional curriculum, which was similar to other PA programs.

In 1971, a significant influence on the subsequent evolution of PA programs came about when the American Medical Association (AMA), along with various collaborating sponsors (American Academy of Family Physicians, American College of Physicians, American Society of Internal Medicine, and American Association of Physicians (AAP)), adopted guidelines for PA program accreditation. These guidelines were published as the *Essentials of an Approved Educational Program for the Assistant to the Primary Care Physician.*

The *Essentials* outlined the criteria upon which program accreditation was based. For the first time, programs would be held accountable for specific aspects of PA education, including institutional sponsorship, curriculum design and sequence, course objectives, faculty qualifications, educational resources and facilities, and ongoing self-study and performance evaluation procedures. Demonstrated compliance with the *Essentials* was required for accreditation by the AMA's Committee on Allied Health Education and Accreditation.

The *Essentials* established minimum standards for all aspects of PA programs. Although they created some uniformity across programs, they allowed for individuality and innovative approaches to PA education. Program accreditation was subsequently incorporated as one of the requirements for seeking federal training grant support.

PA programs have been established in diverse types of sponsoring institutions, including university medical centers, four-year and two-year colleges, public and private hospitals, and branches of the armed services.[9] Institutional sponsorship likely influenced the structure and organization of PA programs, particularly in areas such as admissions policy, faculty and staff appointments, curriculum design and orientation, clinical education, and credential(s) awarded.

For example, currently a PA graduate may earn an associate, baccalaureate, or master's degree, depending on the institution he or she attends. Some may earn a certificate of completion rather than an academic degree. Coincident with variation in the credential awarded, programs have substantial differences in their admission requirements. For example, graduate programs require a baccalaureate degree, while others may require only a high school diploma.

Most programs have a similar curriculum design involving three phases of instruction: basic sciences, introduction to clinical sciences, and supervised clinical instruction. However, programs vary substantially in the amount of time they devote to each phase in the curriculum, the extent of course integration with other students in the health care professions, faculty qualifications and academic level of specific courses, and design of the clinical curriculum. For example, PA students enrolled in programs in medical centers may take courses (including clerkships) with medical students; graduate-level programs may add research-oriented courses to the curriculum, such as statistics, epidemiology, and research design.

The majority of PA programs have traditionally emphasized training in primary care medicine. The federal government helped stimulate this approach by issuing training grant guidelines that established funding preferences for programs emphasizing primary care medicine and utilizing clinical training sites in health manpower shortage areas.[10] The relatively large proportion of PA graduates selecting positions in primary care and locating in health professions shortage areas has been influenced by these federal initiatives.

In addition, the federal government induced programs to respond to important social and educational issues by increasing their minority student enrollments and implementing curricula in geriatric medicine, home health care, AIDS, infant mortality, and preventive medicine. Because PAs take just two years to graduate, the impact of such federal initiatives has been relatively rapid.

The Future of PA Programs
As we pass beyond the 25th anniversary of this profession, PAs will face similar societal and medical issues as those seen in the mid-1960s, such as geographic and specialty maldistribution of physicians and

increasing health care costs. There is general agreement that health care reform in the United States will be implemented within the next few years and will include universal health care coverage and directives for cost containment. As a result, the demand for health care services — and thus the need for primary care providers — will increase substantially.

In addition to fundamental changes in the medical profession, a viable mechanism for responding to the shortage of primary health care providers can be achieved by substantially increasing the number of PAs being trained. In 1992, approximately 1,600 primary care PAs were graduated in the United States. A significantly greater number of PAs could be produced by increasing the number of students admitted to existing programs and establishing more programs. In 1971, when there was a similar shortage of health providers, Congress appropriated funding for the development of additional PA training programs, and within three years 31 new programs were established.[11]

Unlike the 1970s, now we have detailed information on the organization, structure, and outcomes of PA training programs. We can therefore determine whether there are systematic relationships between institutional sponsorship and various characteristics of an educational program, such as:
- the availability of clinical facilities and faculty resources
- levels of financial support and costs of training
- number of applicants and students enrolled
- tuition costs and financial aid available to students
- length and orientation of the curriculum
- and graduate deployment and employment characteristics.

If so, we can determine whether there are inherent advantages to establishing new programs in certain types of institutional settings.

Sources of Information
Physician assistant educational programs in the United States are represented by their national organization, the Association of Physician Assistant Programs (APAP). Since 1984, APAP has sponsored an annual survey of member programs and published the findings as annual reports. Data collected include institutional sponsorship, program budget, curriculum, program personnel, characteristics of applicants, students enrolled, student expenses and attrition, minority representation, and graduate employment information.

Currently (1993), there are 59 AMA-accredited PA programs in the United States, 56 of them primary care and three surgeon's assistant programs. Additional programs are in various stages of development. This paper presents data only on primary care programs. Information on PA curricula was derived from APAP's 1991 *Report;*[12] the remainder of the data were derived from the 1992 *Report.*[13] The response rate to the annual survey has averaged 90 percent since 1984. For some of the data reported here, the number of program respondents to specific items varied, and therefore the totals for a given category may not represent a summation of individual subcategories.

For each of the program characteristics presented, a description of the "typical" PA program will be presented, followed by a comparison of programs on the basis of their institutional sponsorship. Of the 56 primary care PA programs represented, 27 are sponsored by an academic health center (designated as AHC), and 29 are not (designated as non-AHC).

Institutional Sponsorship and Credential Awarded Graduates

The majority of PA programs (83.7 percent) are associated with either a university or a four-year college, and most award graduates either a baccalaureate (62.5 percent) or master's degree (16 percent) on completion. The remainder are associated with a two-year college (awarding an associate of arts or science degree) or are hospital-based. All programs award graduates a certificate of completion, the minimum credential required for registering for the National Certifying Examination.

The administrative organization of PA programs within the sponsoring institution varies widely. Most programs are affiliated with a college of medicine or schools of associated medical sciences, health professions, or allied health sciences. Within these domains, some programs have departmental status, some are organized as divisions, and others are defined as educational units within a department, typically in family medicine, primary care medicine, or community medicine.

PA programs also have external affiliations with a variety of clinical facilities where the majority of supervised clinical instruction occurs. These sites include tertiary care medical centers, public and private teaching hospitals, health maintenance organizations, and veterans administration medical centers or hospitals. In addition, programs typically have an extensive network of community-based clinical teaching sites in single- and multi-specialty clinics and office practices. The clinical faculty are practicing physicians (and PAs) who may not have appointments within the sponsoring institution.

The highest credential awarded graduates is shown in Table 1. In both AHC-sponsored and non-AHC programs, the majority of students receive a baccalaureate degree (56 percent and 69 percent, respectively). In recent years, nine PA programs have converted from a baccalaureate- to a graduate-level curriculum, the majority (67 percent; N=6) of which are associated with AHCs. The master's programs, data of conversion and sponsorship status are as follows (an asterisk denotes AHC sponsorship):

- University of Colorado (1974)*
- Northeastern University (1984)
- Emory University (1988)*
- Baylor University (1990)*
- Duke University (1990)*
- University of Iowa (1992)*
- University of Nebraska (1992)*
- University of Detroit Mercy (1992)
- Duquesne University (1992)

It is anticipated that additional programs will convert to a graduate-level curriculum over the next few years, and most will be AHC-sponsored. Although most programs offer an academic degree, a few (N=6) award graduates a certificate of completion as the highest credential, and most of these are located in an academic health center.

Table 1
Credentials Earned on Graduation

Credential Earned	AHC-Sponsored		Non-AHC-Sponsored	
	N	(%)	N	(%)
Certificate Only	4	14.8%	2	6.9%
Associate (AA/AS)	2	7.4%	4	13.8%
Baccalaureate	15	55.6%	20	69.0%
Master's	6	22.2%	3	10.3%
Total	27		29	

PA Program Budgets

For the 1991-92 academic year, the typical PA program reported a total budget of $470,000, derived from a varying combination of sources, including the sponsoring institution, student tuition and fees, federal training grants, and state grants. Most programs received the majority of their funding from two sources: the sponsoring institution and federal training grants. Seventy-seven percent of the programs reported receiving federal grants, which averaged $129,000 per program.

Regarding program budget, respondents reported the amount and source of *direct* financial support. In the main, this included salaries for core faculty and support staff and funds for general expenses. Core personnel were defined as individuals who devoted more than 50 percent of their time to program activities. Thus, costs associated with non-PA program faculty or staff who may provide educational and/or support services to the program were typically *not* included in the budget figures. For example, some faculty members within the institution or clinical preceptors external to the institution may not have received *direct* reimbursement from the program but provided services without financial compensation or were funded by the institution.

Table 2 compares the budgets of AHC-sponsored and non-AHC programs. The total budget for AHC-sponsored programs was 12 percent higher ($51,100) than non-AHC programs. In addition, twice as many AHC programs (N=25; mean=$139,708) received support from federal training grants as did non-AHC programs (N=12; mean=$109,167). On average, grant support accounted for 30 percent and 26 percent of the program budget, respectively. PA training grants are awarded by the Division of Medicine in the Health Re-

Table 2
Program Budget and Student Expenses

Characteristic	AHC-Sponsored		Non-AHC-Sponsored	
	Mean	SD	Mean	SD
Total Program Budget	$ 473,700	$ 220,000	$ 422,600	$ 210,000
Fed. PA Grants*	$ 139,708	$ 90,002	$ 109,167	$ 63,000
Percent of Budget	29.5%		25.8%	
Cost per Student	$ 8,029	N/A	$ 7,546	N/A

*25 AHC programs and 12 Non-AHC programs

sources and Services Administration's Bureau of Health Professions and are typically on a three-year, competitive application cycle. As mentioned, the Division established funding priorities in specific areas, and programs must address these preferences to remain competitive for grant support.

During the 1991-92 academic year, total enrollment averaged 59 students in AHC-sponsored and 56 students in non-AHC programs (see Table 5). Given the figures for the program budget and total student enrollment, the cost of training a PA student can be approximated. Thus, for AHC-sponsored programs, the estimated cost of training a PA over two years was $16,058 per student, while that of non-AHC programs was $15,092 per student, a 6 percent difference.

These figures are rough estimates and do not include all forms of support from the institution. For example, a faculty member appointed and receiving salary from the department of biochemistry may teach biochemistry for PA students, a service for which the PA program does not pay. Similarly, a clinical preceptor at an external site providing clinical education to a PA student may serve without compensation, receiving a salary from the affiliate. In either case, the PA program would not report the monetary value of these educational services as a part of the program budget.

Lastly, the program's overhead costs may not be factored into reported budget figures. Some programs, however, reimburse both didactic and clinical faculty for their services, and these figures are typically reported.

Student Expenses

The typical resident PA student admitted in 1991 paid $13,890 for tuition, books, fees, and equipment during two years of enrollment; the non-resident student paid $18,440. Tuition accounted for the majority (86 percent) of these costs.

As shown in Table 3, resident students enrolled in AHC-sponsored programs had substantially lower educational costs (31 percent or $3,800 less) than did those enrolled in non-AHC programs. There was less of a difference between the two groups (5 percent or $900) in the costs for the non-resident student. Proportionately, there were more non-AHC programs associated with private schools (with higher tuition rates). In addition, resident and non-resident tuition in private schools is usually the same.

Table 3
Student Expenses

Characteristic	AHC-Sponsored		Non-AHC-Sponsored	
	Mean	SD	Mean	SD
Tuition/Books/Fees*				
Resident	$ 12,200	$ 7,210	$ 16,000	$ 7,970
Non-Resident	$ 19,100	$ 8,110	$ 18,000	$ 6,450
Financial Aid				
Amt Received*	$ 14,360	$ 4,300	$ 13,560	$ 4,510
% Receiving	71.5%	19.0	71.4%	22.9

*For Entire Professional Program (24 months)

The majority of PA students received financial aid in 1991, and the proportion did not differ on the basis of program sponsorship. Ostensibly, the remaining students financed their PA education through savings or parental and/or spousal assistance. The typical student enrolled in an AHC-sponsored program received 5 percent more financial aid than students enrolled in non-AHC programs. It appears that the amount of financial aid received was nearly equal to the expenses associated with the student's tuition, books, and fees.

Based on these financial aid figures, it can be estimated that the majority (71 percent) of students will have a debt of approximately $13,500 to $14,500 at the conclusion of their professional education. This debt does not include the costs of students' pre-PA education or the costs associated with room and board and incidental expenses while in the program.

The Applicant Pool and PA Student Enrollment
In 1991, the typical program received 134 applications and reported a ratio of four applicants for each student enrolled. The average size of the first-year PA class was 32.2 students, 60 percent of whom were women. Twenty percent were ethnic minorities, predominantly African-Americans.

The total first-year enrollment was 1,771 students, of which 6 percent were enrolled on a part-time basis. On average, 4 percent of the maximum capacity of the first-year class remained unfilled. The second-year class averaged 27.0 students per program. Thus, in 1991 total enrollment across all PA programs was estimated to be 3,408 (322 more students than the previous year). The attrition rate across all programs averaged 8.7 percent.

Interest in the PA profession has increased substantially over the past five years, as evidenced by increases in the applicant pool. Table 4 shows the number of applicants and students enrolled in PA programs from 1988 through 1992. During this period, the number of applicants increased by 136 percent, and enrollment increased by 37 percent.

As shown in Table 5, the ratio of applicants to first-year enrollment in 1991-92 for AHC-sponsored and non-AHC programs was 4:1 and was similar between the two groups. However, the total number

---

Table 4
Applicants and Students Enrolled: 1988-1992

Academic Year	Applicants Programs	First Year Enrollment	Annual Increase
1988-89	86.1	25.9	-
1989-90	90.2	26.1	4.8%
1990-91	106.5	29.6	18.0%
1991-92	133.2	32.2	25.1%
1992-93	203.0	35.0	52.4%

*Drawn from the 1993 APAP Survey, unpublished.

Table 5
Applicants and Students Enrolled: 1991-92

Applicants/Enrollment	AHC-Sponsored		Non-AHC-Sponsored	
	Mean	SD	Mean	SD
Total Applicants	140.1	49.5	124.4	51.4
Total Enrollment	59.4	18.9	55.6	15.8
Characteristics:				
First-Year Class	34.3	7.1	29.9	8.1
Non-Minority	80.5%	N/A	80.9%	N/A
Minority	19.5%	N/A	19.1%	N/A
Ratio (Appl/1st year)	4:1	N/A	4:1	N/A
Attrition Rate	8.8%	N/A	8.7%	N/A

of applicants and enrollment of the first-year class differed; there were an average of 13 percent more applicants (N=15.7) and students enrolled (N=4.4) in AHC-sponsored programs compared to non-AHC programs.

The proportion of minority students was comparable between the two groups, as were program attrition rates. Attrition from all PA programs occurred primarily during the first year and was reported to be primarily due to academic (55 percent) and personal reasons (37 percent, includes financial and health problems).

Admission Requirements

The typical PA program's prerequisites include a minimum of two years of college-level preparatory courses in general liberal arts studies and specific courses in the natural and physical sciences (biology, chemistry, mathematics and/or physics). As noted earlier, a majority of PA programs enroll students who had already completed a baccalaureate degree irrespective of the degree granted by the program. For example, it has been reported that more than 50 percent of the students enrolled in the community college or hospital-based programs had earned a baccalaureate degree prior to admission![14]

Most programs have implemented two other requirements: health-related experience (preferably with direct patient contact) and a pre-admission interview to ascertain the candidate's interpersonal and communications skills, motivation for pursuing a clinical career, and rationale for selecting the PA profession. A positive correlation has been demonstrated between pre-admission interview ratings and subsequent *clinical* performance.[15]

In 1991, the typical entering student could be described as a white female over 26 years of age, with a grade point average of 3.10 and more than four years of health care experience prior to admission. Most students were residents of the state in which their program was located.

Some master's-level programs require different prerequisites, usually a baccalaureate degree and scores on national examinations (Graduate Record Exam and/or Medical College Admission Tests). In some cases, programs have identified research-related requirements, such as prior research experience or specific course requirements (e.g., statistics).

Curriculum

PA educators responsible for developing a curriculum were rather innovative, by both design and default. Given a relatively brief time to prepare students for the practice of medicine, they had to revise existing courses or create new ones; they also had to identify an essential body of knowledge and dispense with whatever was extraneous. In addition, programs actively pursued innovative instructional and evaluation techniques. These have included: using simulated patients and videotapes to assess interviewing and physical examination skills; adopting problem-oriented approaches to didactic instruction; using clinical vignettes for assessing physical examination competencies; and incorporating patient management problems for evaluating data management and problem-solving skills.

The typical PA curriculum averages two years (98 weeks) in length, but length varies extensively across programs (range of 52 to 156 weeks). The curriculum is similar in sequence to that of the traditional medical school model:

- Phase I: basic medical sciences (and behavioral sciences)
- Phase II: introductory clinical medicine
- Phase III: rotating clinical clerkships or rotations

Typically, Phases I and II comprise the first year and Phase III the second year of the curriculum.

The data reported in this section were drawn from the 1990 survey of PA programs.[16] Respondents were asked to provide the hours and weeks of instruction associated with the didactic and clinical phases of their program. Although there was considerable variation across programs, a core curriculum was identified, based on whether a majority (>50 percent) of programs reported they had a particular course or clinical rotation in their curriculum.

Overall, the total length of the curriculum of AHC-sponsored programs was nearly four weeks longer (mean=99.8 weeks) than the non-AHC program curriculum (mean=96.0 weeks). Table 6 identifies the hours of instruction associated with the first year of the curriculum for the two groups of programs. Relative to Phase I, programs sponsored by AHCs had devoted approximately 57 more hours (12 percent increase) of instruction in the basic and behavioral sciences (N=544 hours) than the non-AHC programs (N=487). The difference in hours of basic science instruction was principally in three courses: anatomy (+22 hours), physiology (+18 hours), and

Table 6
Pre-Clinical Curriculum

Hours of Instruction*	AHC-Sponsored		Non-AHC	
	Mean	SD	Mean	SD
Phase I:				
Basic Science	407.6	176.0	386.2	136.0
Beh Sci/Prof Issues	135.3	100.3	100.3	61.1
Sub-Total	543.9	N/A	486.5	N/A
Phase II:				
Didactic Clin. Med.	300.5	174.4	269.7	122.8
Patient Assessment	143.3	51.7	119.8	30.1
Interviewing (Hx)	45.8	N/A	35.9	N/A
Phys. Exam (Px)	97.5	N/A	83.9	N/A
Technical Skills	41.0	36.0	38.8	29.9
Sub-Total	484.8		428.3	
Phase I + II: Total	1027.7	327.9	914.8	221.6

*Includes lecture, laboratory, and discussion.

biochemistry (+12 hours). The behavioral science curriculum included courses such as psychosocial dynamics, health promotion, health care organization, professional issues, human sexuality and medical ethics. As there was considerable variation in the values given, the significance of any differences is difficult to define. On average, Phase I of the curriculum was six to seven months in length.

Phase II of the typical program involved approximately five to six months of instruction and included three types of educational activity: didactic clinical instruction, patient assessment, and technical skills. In each of these categories, the AHC-sponsored programs provided more hours of instruction than the non-AHC programs, a 13-percent difference. In some programs, Phases I and II were extensively integrated, while in other programs they were discrete elements. Technical skills included instruction in cardiopulmonary resuscitation, assisted cardiopulmonary life support, casting, suturing, and injection.

In summary, for the first-year curriculum, programs in academic health centers reported a total of 1,028 hours of instruction as compared to 915 hours for the non-AHC programs, an overall difference of 113 hours of instruction (12 percent).

A Unique Model for the Clinical Curriculum

The organization and management of clinical instruction in PA programs typically involves a rotational, outreach approach. PA programs have developed clinical affiliations with hospitals, clinics, and office-based practices that are separate and often distant from the sponsoring institution. For example, programs associated with a medical school may have very few rotations at the medical center, and these rotations would typically be in specialty and sub-specialty areas of medicine. The bulk of the clinical instruction would occur externally at a number of affiliated sites. These external sites may range from inner-city clinics to rural satellite facilities.

Some programs have developed an end-of-program preceptorship, whereby students are placed at a clinical site (usually in a primary care specialty) that also has the potential to become an employment opportunity with the supervising physician. In certain instances, the preceptors may have been identified and recruited by the student prior to admission to the program. The concept of coupling a student's clinical training with employment on graduation is indicative of those programs that have adopted the Medex model of education. Obviously, such an approach increases the probability that a graduate will seek employment in primary care medicine, often in a health professions shortage area.

The rationale for adopting an outreach approach to clinical education is two-fold. First, it provides the student with the opportunity to have contact with ambulatory patients in a primary care setting which more closely simulates the clinical environment in which most PA graduates will find themselves. Second, completing rotations external to the medical center reduces the competition the PA student would have for patient care experience with medical students, residents, and fellows.

Another advantage to such an approach is that programs have made an effort to develop clinical affiliations with facilities that also employ graduate PAs. As such, these individuals (referred to as staff or on-site PAs) will serve as role models and mentors to the student. In addition, they may assist with the orientation, education, and evaluation of PA students.

Although the outreach model is an effective method of providing students with an appropriate clinical education and opportunity for role identification, it entails special administrative and resource needs. For example, additional personnel are required to develop, schedule and monitor external clinical sites on a continuous basis. There are also attendant requirements for supporting student travel and housing accommodations. Lastly, this model requires students to assume a proactive role and substantial responsibility for their education; they are not subject to direct supervision by program faculty, as is the case during the first year of the curriculum.

Supervised Clinical Instruction

The typical PA program provides 51.5 weeks of instruction in supervised clinical education in both primary care and non-primary care medical specialties. The typical PA student will complete 34.9 weeks of instruction in primary care medicine and 16.6 weeks in non-primary care medicine. As discussed above, the clinical education of PAs generally occurs external to the sponsoring institution.

A comparison and general summary of the clinical curriculum for students matriculating through AHC versus non-AHC programs is shown in Table 7. On average, the clinical curriculum associated with the AHC-sponsored programs was 3.2 weeks longer than non-AHC programs. Proportionately, the students in AHC-sponsored programs spent more time during their clinical year in primary care medical specialties (70 percent) than did students in non-AHC programs (67 percent). As will be discussed in the following section, the graduate's selection of a primary care specialty and deployment to underserved areas may be influenced by similar experiences while he or she is a student in training.

The greater student involvement in primary care instruction

Table 7
Clinical Curriculum

Weeks of Instruction	AHC-Sponsored		Non-AHC-Sponsored	
	Mean	SD	Mean	SD
Total Length	52.3	8.5	49.1	7.6
Primary Care	36.4	10.1	33.0	4.9
Non-Primary Care	15.9	7.8	16.1	6.9

among AHC-sponsored programs may be related to the fact that twice the number of these programs receive federal support (see Table 2). Recall that one of the priorities for the PA training grants was that programs must demonstrate that students will have clinical experience in primary care medicine and at sites situated in medically underserved areas. The federal training grants include opportunities to apply for funds that can be used to identify and recruit primary care preceptors and provide students with travel support and housing.

PA Program Graduates

The average size of the 1991 graduating class was 23.1 students. Fifty-four percent were employed in primary care specialties, principally family or general internal medicine. The most common non-primary care specialties selected by recent graduates were surgery (especially cardiovascular and cardiothoracic surgery) and the internal medicine subspecialties, typically cardiology.

The demand for 1991 graduates greatly exceeds supply, with a ratio of 6.2 employment opportunities for each recent graduate. The majority (88 percent) of new graduates were employed within 20.2 weeks of graduation. Starting salaries continue to increase annually, averaging $36,815 in 1991, 2.7 percent above that in 1990 ($35,856).

In total, the typical program has graduated 17 classes and matriculated 384 students. It is estimated that over 85 percent of all PAs are employed in a clinical position and a majority (53 percent) are employed in a primary care medical specialty in either an office (35 percent) or hospital setting (33 percent). These physician assistants are typically employed in either family medicine (32 percent), generally internal medicine (11 percent), or in a surgical subspecialty (11 percent). In 1976, approximately 75 percent of PAs were employed in primary care.

A comparison of the employment characteristics of recent (1991) and all PA graduates from AHC-sponsored or non-AHC programs is presented in Table 8. Although the total number of recent graduates did not differ between the two groups (means of 23.0 and 23.4 students per program), the proportion of these graduates selecting a primary care position for their first employment differed by approximately 8 percent, with AHC program graduates more likely to be so employed than non-AHC program graduates. It may very well be that the observed difference in selection of primary care medical special-

Table 8
Graduates and Type of Practice

Graduate Employment	AHC-Sponsored		Non-AHC-Sponsored	
	Mean	SD	Mean	SD
Number Recent Graduates*	23.4	8.6	23.0	8.5
% in Primary Care	57.6%	N/A	49.7%	N/A
Total Number Graduates*	271.4	108.1	253.1	119.3
% in Primary Care	54.1%	N/A	52.5%	N/A

*Employed in a Clinical Position

ties among AHC-sponsored programs was due to the fact that the students spent more time in primary care specialties during their clinical curriculum. It has been fairly well documented that there is a relationship between third-year medical student clerkships in family medicine and graduating students' choice of family practice careers.[17] This relationship likely also applies to PA students.

There were more PA graduates from the AHC programs (N=271) than those graduating from non-AHC programs (N=253). However, the proportion of the total graduates employed in primary care medical specialties did not differ substantially between the two groups.

Certification of PA Graduates

PAs achieve certification by passing an entry-level, National Certifying Examination prepared by the National Board of Medical Examiners and administered by the National Commission on Certification of Physician Assistants (NCCPA). Graduation (certificate) from an AMA-approved program is required to be eligible to sit for the examination.

The two-day examination consists of a multiple choice core component (3.5 hours), a specialty multiple choice component (2.5 hours) in either primary care or surgery and a practical exam of clinical skills. The performance of program graduates sitting for the 1992 Physician Assistant National Certifying Examination is shown in Table 9. The data were drawn from the 1992 NCCPA report to PA programs and include the mean, standard error of measurement, median and range of scores across all PA programs with five or more examinees. In 1992, 2,121 examinees from 55 PA programs were

Table 9
Scores on the 1992 National Certifying Examination

Exam Component	Program Mean	SEM	Median	Range of Scores	Minimum Pass
Core Objective	499	30	505	375-630	410
Primary Care	478	37	480	365-600	300
Surgery	484	40	485	370-570	300
CSP	481	57	480	380-585	300

represented; 1,531 were recent graduates. The pass rate for all examinees was 76 percent; for those classified as first takers (recent graduates) the pass rate was higher (85 percent). As indicated in Table 9, there was a relatively large range in the mean scores of programs, especially in the core objective exam. The minimum pass level also differed between the core objective exam and either of the three remaining exams.

To become certified, a candidate must pass both the core and clinical skills practice exam and either the primary care or surgery exams. A successful examinee is designated a PA-C, and certification is required in most states (N=42) for a PA to practice. In 1992, 1,605 examinees were certified; a total of 24,355 examinees have been certified since 1974.

Selected Comparisons between Medical and PA Students
During the 1991-92 academic year, 17,027 medical students were admitted to the 126 medical schools in the United States,[18] a figure nearly 11-fold greater than the number of PA students enrolled in 56 PA programs. The ratio of medical school applicants to students enrolled was 1.9:1, compared to a 4:1 ratio among PA applicants and students enrolled. Attrition from medical school has been relatively low (1.3 percent) and due principally to poor academic performance (36 percent), transfer to another institution (25 percent), and personal problems (21 percent, including financial and health). Although the reasons for attrition are similar for PA students, the rate of attrition is nearly seven-fold higher (8.7 percent in 1991) than for medical students.

The proportion of minority students entering medical school has remained relatively unchanged over the past decade at approximately

10 percent per year,[19] a figure approximately one-half that of PA programs, which have averaged 21.5 percent minority enrollment over the past nine years.[20] It has been shown that minority physicians tend to practice more frequently in minority underserved locations than do majority physicians,[21] a relationship which also holds for PAs.

Median tuition for first-year medical students attending private medical schools in 1991 was $18,930 per year. Resident students attending public medical schools had a median tuition of $6,115 and for nonresident students, $13,839 per year.[22] For the same academic year (1990-91), tuition for students enrolled in PA programs was substantially lower than for medical students, $5,310 for resident students and $7,307 for nonresident students.[23] Unfortunately, data comparing tuition for private and public PA schools are not available.

The mean educational debt for the typical medical student in 1991 was estimated to be $50,884 with 78 percent of medical school graduates indebted for that year.[24] Although a similar proportion (71 percent) of PA students incur debt at the completion of their education, their debt is approximately one-third as great ($13,500-$14,500).

Summary of Findings

The data presented here suggest that establishing PA programs in academic health centers may have some advantages, such as:

- lower program and student costs
- a larger applicant pool and enrollment
- a longer curriculum with more emphasis on primary care training
- and a larger proportion of graduates employed as generalists.

However, these differences were relatively modest. In addition, the variation across programs in each of these categories was relatively large. Thus, one must be cautious in making specific recommendations concerning the type of institution which would be best suited for establishing PA programs.

Responding to the Need for Primary Care Providers

It is estimated that 80 percent of contacts that patients have with physicians could be effectively managed by primary care physicians and at least 70 percent of these patients could be capably handled by physician assistants.

Although it is generally acknowledged that for the optimal delivery of health care in the United States over half of all physicians should be in primary care, currently, nearly 70 percent are practicing as specialists.[25] Further, more medical graduates are selecting residency training in specialties versus primary care. For example, in 1992, only 14.6 percent of graduating seniors opted for primary care specialties (family medicine, 9 percent, general internal medicine, 3.2 percent, and general pediatrics, 2.4 percent), a decrease from 36 percent in 1982.[26] Conversely, more than 50 percent of PAs are practicing in primary care, and a similar proportion of new graduates are selecting practice as generalists each year.[27]

It has been well documented that physician specialists providing primary care add to the costs of medical care delivery, including the care provided to Medicare recipients.[28] Specialists order more diagnostic tests, perform more procedures and hospitalize more patients than primary care physicians treating a similar mix of patients. In addition, the salaries of specialist physicians are considerably higher than those of primary care doctors. In 1989, the mean salaries for surgical and medical specialists were $220,500 and $146,500, respectively, while salaries for generalists averaged $95,900.[29]

A Complementary Approach to Resolving the Problem

To date, most discussion surrounding the issue of resolving the primary health care crisis has focused on strategies to increase the production of physician generalists and improve their practice situation. This approach is very complex and would involve major changes in a variety of areas, including medical student and faculty attitudes, medical school curricula, physician clinical behaviors, Medicare reimbursement policy, and distribution of medical expenditures across specialties.[30]

Indeed, the Association of American Medical Colleges has recently set forth a series of comprehensive recommendations directed to schools of medicine, graduate medical education, and the practice environment, with a general policy statement advocating a national goal that a "majority of graduating medical students be committed to generalist careers...."[31] However, it is not at all certain that these efforts will be implemented in the near future; nor is it clear that they would solve the problem. Even under the most optimistic course of events, given the length of time required to produce physician generalists (a minimum of seven years), improvements in the generalist/

specialist ratio of physicians could not be realized until after the year 2000.

In addition to these initiatives, compelling data support the notion that PAs may offer a complementary and realistic approach to resolving the health care crisis, at least in the short term. First, on average, it takes two years of professional training to prepare a PA for clinical practice; the majority will enter primary care specialties. Given the substantial size of the applicant pool and demonstrated interest in this profession, the annual production of PAs could be increased four-fold within two to three years if additional resources were available to increase enrollment and establish additional programs. The latter could most effectively be accomplished by decreasing medical student enrollment and utilizing the resultant release of faculty, financial, and physical resources to create additional PA educational programs in schools of medicine.

Second, as PAs practice in a fashion similar to that of primary care physicians in terms of their clinical behaviors (i.e., frequency of ordering laboratory tests, performing procedures, and recommending hospitalization) they offer the prospects of significant reductions in health care costs. These financial benefits are further enhanced because PAs earn approximately one-third the income of generalist physicians while working a similar number of hours per week and weeks per year, and they can effectively manage the majority of patients visiting a primary care practice.[32] In this regard, appropriate changes would need to be made in Medicare policy to extend reimbursement of PA services to PAs located in office-based practices. In addition, as only 33 states permit PAs to write prescriptions, it would be necessary to effect legislation to extend these privileges in the remaining states in order to optimize PA practice activities.

References

1. Hudson CL. Expansion of medical professional services with nonprofessional personnel. *JAMA.* 1961;176:839-41. Brown NS, Jacobziner H, Becker H. Closing the gaps in the availability and accessibility of health services: introductory remarks. *Bull NY Acad Med.* 1965;41:1197-1212. Stead EA. Conserving costly talents: providing physicians new assistants. *JAMA.* 1966;198:182-3. Stead EA Jr. Educational programs and manpower. *Bull NY Acad Med.* 1968;44:204-213.
2. Perry HB. An analysis of the professional performance of physician assistants. *JME.* 1977;52:639-647. Duttera MJ, Harlan WR. Evaluation of physician assistants in rural primary care. *Arch Int Med.* 1978;138:224-228.
3. Record JC. *Staffing Primary Care in 1990: Physician Replacement and Cost Savings.* New York: Springer

Publishing Company; 1981:68-84. Carter RD, Perry HB, Oliver DR. *Secondary Analysis: The 1981 National Survey of Physician Assistants, Methodology and Findings on Productivity.* Alexandria, Va: Association of Physician Assistant Programs; 1984.

4. Record JC, McCally M, Schweitzer SO, et al. New health professionals after a decade and a half: delegation, productivity and costs in primary care. *J Health Policy.* 1980;5:470-496.
5. Stead EA. Training and use of paramedical personnel. *N Engl J Med.* 1967;277:800-2.
6. Smith RA. MEDEX. *JAMA.* 1970;211:1843-5.
7. Silver HK, Ford LC, Day LR. The pediatric nurse-practitioner program. *JAMA.* 1968;204:298-302.
8. Myers JC. The physician assistant in community hospital and office practice. *NY Acad Sci.* 1968;166:911-5.
9. Association of Physician Assistant Programs. *Programs Directory.* Alexandria, Va; 1992.
10. Bureau of Health Professions. *Health Resources and Services Administrative Annual Report: Grants for Programs for Physician Assistants.* Rockville, Md: Health Resources and Services Administration; 1990.
11. Oliver DR, Conboy J, Donahue W, McKelvey P. Survey of physician's assistant programs in the United States. *J Med Ed.* 1986;61:757-760.
12. Oliver DR, Baker J. *Seventh Annual Report on Physician Assistant Educational Programs in the United States, 1990-91.* Alexandria, Va: Association of Physician Assistant Programs; 1991.
13. Oliver DR, Baker J. *Eighth Annual Report on Physician Assistant Educational Programs in the United States, 1991-92.* Alexandria, Va: Association of Physician Assistant Programs; 1992.
14. Oliver DR, Baker J. *Seventh Annual Report on Physician Assistant Educational Programs in the United States, 1990-91.* Alexandria, Va: Association of Physician Assistant Programs; 1991.
15. Oliver DR, Preston M, Bratton B. An analysis of the relationship among selection factors, program and professional achievement of physician assistants. Presentation to the Association of Physician Assistant Programs; May 5, 1980; New Orleans, La.
16. Oliver DR, Baker J. *Seventh Annual Report on Physician Assistant Educational Programs in the United States, 1990-91.* Alexandria, Va: Association of Physician Assistant Programs; 1991.
17. Kassebaum D, Haynes R. Relationship between third-year clerkships in family medicine and graduating students' choice of family practice careers. *Acad Med.* 1992;67:217-219.
18. Jonas HS, Etzel S, Barzansky B. Educational programs in U.S. medical schools. *JAMA.* 1992;268:1063-1090.
19. Association of American Medical Colleges. *Minority Students in Medical Education: Facts and Figures VI.* Washington, DC: Association of American Medical Colleges; 1991.
20. Oliver DR, Baker J. *Eighth Annual Report on Physician Assistant Educational Programs in the United States, 1991-92.* Alexandria, Va: Association of Physician Assistant Programs; 1992.
21. Satcher D. Barriers to equity in access for racial/ethnic minorities. In: *Education of Physicians to Improve Access to Care for the Underserved: Proceedings from the Second HRSA Primary Care Conference, March 21-23, 1990.* Rockville, Md: Health Resources and Services Administration; 1991.
22. Jolly P, Hudley D, eds. *AAMC Data Book.* U.S. schools of median tuition and fees. Washington, DC: Association of American Medical Colleges; July, 1991.
23. Oliver DR, Baker J. *Seventh Annual Report on Physician Assistant Educational Programs in the United States, 1990-91.* Alexandria, Va: Association of Physician Assistant Programs; 1991.
24. Association of American Medical Colleges. *Financing a Medical Education in the '90s: Collective Concerns — Paying the Bills and Preventing Defaults. A report of the Committee on Student Financial Assistance.* Washington, DC: Association of American Medical Colleges; 1991.
25. Council on Graduate Medical Education. *Third Report: Improving Access to Health Care Through Physician Workforce Reform: Directions for the 21st Century.* Rockville, Md: Health Resources and Services Administration; 1992.
26. Kassebaum DG, Szenas PL. Relationship between indebtedness and the specialty choices of graduating medical students. *Acad Med.* 1992;67:700-7.
27. Oliver DR, Baker J. *Eighth Annual Report on Physician Assistant Educational Programs in the United States, 1991-92.* Alexandria, Va: Association of Physician Assistant Programs; 1992.
28. Greenfield S, Nelson EC, Zubkoff M, et al. Variations in resource utilization among medical specialties and systems of care: results from the Medical Outcomes Study. *JAMA.* 1992;267:1624-30. Welch WP, Miller ME, Welch HG, Fisher ES, Wennberg JE. Geographic variation in expenditures for physicians' services in the United States. *N Engl J Med.* 1993;328:621-7.
29. Pope GC, Schneider JE. Trends in physician income. *Health Affairs.* 1992;11:181-193.
30. Kassirer JP. Primary care and the affliction of internal medicine. *N Engl J Med.* 1993;328:649-651. Petersdorf RG. Financing medical education - a universal "Berry Plan" for medical students. *N Engl*

J Med. 1993;328:651-654. Fitzgerald, FT. The case for internal medicine. *N Engl J Med.* 1993; 328:654-6. Levinsky NG. Recruiting for primary care. *N Engl J Med.* 1993;328:656-660.

31. Association of American Medical Colleges Task Force on the Generalist Physician. Strategy Statement on the Generalist Physician. Washington, DC: Association of American Medical Colleges; 1992.

32. Carter RD, Perry HP, Oliver DR. *Secondary Analysis: the 1981 National Survey of Physician Assistants, Methodology and Findings on Productivity.* Alexandria, Va: Association of Physician Assistant Programs; 1984.

8

Training Doctors for the Future: Lessons from 25 Years of Physician Assistant Education

E. Harvey Estes, Jr.

IN 25 YEARS OF EXPERIENCE WITH PHYSICIAN ASSISTANT education, I have gleaned many lessons.[1] Three of the most significant are:

1. An innovation addressing a societal need has a very high probability of becoming an accepted and established component of society.
2. A responsible individual whose performance is continuously reviewed and judged by peers is a more reliable guarantor of performance than an administrative system relying on credentials, rules, and regulations.
3. The educational system producing physician assistants is more advanced, efficient, and cost-effective than that producing physicians.

The Importance of Meeting Societal Needs

All human systems are driven and molded by the system of rewards that provides the incentives and disincentives for the individuals within the system. These rewards can be of many types, such as higher pay, political power, or esteem of others. Most of the time, they are a mixture. Money, power, and esteem tend to track together, with money being the most convenient proxy for the entire reward system.

However, money and esteem may diverge, as is often seen in the practice of medicine. A rural practitioner may receive high levels of esteem and little money, and a "fashionable" plastic surgeon may receive very high pay but little public warmth. Each responds to his or her rewards by working harder to gain more, and each probably views his or her rewards as better than the other's.

Over the past 25 years, medical centers and medical schools have been distorted by a reward system that has overvalued research and new technological advances and undervalued the production of graduates to meet the recognized medical needs of average people. The unprecedented investment of public funds through the National Institutes of Health and the high payment awarded for new technologies have brought money and fame to certain medical school faculty and graduates. These trends have distorted the character of teaching and influenced the choice of careers among students.

This distortion was evident in the 1950s and '60s but did not evoke much professional or public reaction. Practitioners in community practice largely were content with their lot until the medical centers were no longer able to supply their replacements. At that point, overwork and burnout — not inadequate payment —began to force them out of practice, leaving human needs unmet and causing those with unmet needs to call for answers. Consequently, in the late 1960s and early 1970s, society forced many changes upon the medical education system, a system which did not recognize its own role in causing these changes.

The physician assistant (PA) concept grew out of an effort to assist and replace practitioners who had been serving the medical needs of people primarily in underserved areas. The concept was quickly accepted because it met a real need. PAs were restricted by a requirement that they be supervised by physicians. This restriction inhibited their dispersion and flexibility to a degree, but it had the advantage of providing a link to a source of care with which patients were familiar.

In the 1960s, an unhappy society mandated a sharp increase in the number of medical students being trained. By the late 1970s, concern was growing in the medical profession that there might be too many physicians in the near future. Many proposed that physician assistant programs be shut down, because the expected excess of physicians would make them superfluous.

At that time, another social need arose, and again the midlevel practitioner provided an answer. Rising costs in medical care became a major issue, and an urgent need to provide care at lower cost emerged. This need was not restricted to those areas with no providers; it existed in all areas of medicine. Specialists, including those in academic medical centers, finding that they needed skilled help in performing defined portions of their services, turned to midlevel practitioners to meet these needs.

Social needs, unmet by the medical profession, have allowed a new group of practitioners to become quickly established and accepted as a member of the health professional community. This group often shares the public esteem and the other non-financial rewards of medical practice to a degree equal to the physician.

The physician community has, through its lack of attention to the needs of major segments of society, allowed a potential competitor to enter the field. For most physicians, this competition is not currently a problem, because the supervisory role of the physician is established in law in most states, and payment is to the physician-midlevel team, not to the midlevel practitioner alone. Also, a physician-midlevel practitioner team can earn sufficient added income, above that of the physician alone, to more than pay the added salary of the midlevel.

However, it is vital to remember that the current system is based on today's set of rewards. If the tide of public funding for the research enterprise is reduced, if payment for highly technical procedures is more closely aligned with payment for less technical procedures, and if more physicians enter primary care practices, we may find that much of the public will prefer a midlevel practitioner instead of a physician and that financial rewards will follow.

I believe that this situation will come to pass in many rural areas of the country. Fortunately, the roots of medical education and PA education are sufficiently commingled that these professions can work together, and I believe that they will do so, probably to the benefit of both.

On the other hand, the nursing profession is following the same path that medicine has followed over the past half century, and it may fall into the same trap. Instead of emphasizing the rewards of patient care and service to people, the profession is emphasizing academic degrees, research, and autonomy. Nursing educators should put their faith in the social need for NPs as a source of justification and authority — and move to meet that need — instead of relying on research skills and degrees. They should also seek to gain as much as possible from their working relationship with physicians, including commingled education, instead of building walls around their profession and turning aside the willingness of physicians to assist them in training the most competent practitioner possible. Medicine and nursing have too much to learn from each other to stand apart.

It is also clear that society would be best served by a generalist midlevel practitioner, prepared to serve the unfiltered problems of those who are in the most severe need, rather than an assortment of specialized, compartmentalized practitioners. The PA profession has always, with a few exceptions, produced a generally trained graduate, while nursing has tended to favor specialty-specific training. The discipline should reassess its directions to meet the needs of those it serves.

Training Physicians To Supervise Staff

Physician assistants develop their practice style and content by a process of negotiated delegation with the supervising physician. This has proved to be a fairly good system, but it has some deficiencies, largely relating to the fact that physicians are not trained to supervise and to function as the leader of a team serving the patient. Whether a given practice employs a midlevel practitioner or not, the physician is the leader of a large team of individuals who are essential for the proper care of the patient.

The person who answers the telephone and serves as the principal interface with patients is one of the most important people in the team, and the physician should be sure that patient access is pleasant and easy. The billing clerk is equally important. Most patients are confused and helpless with respect to the payment system, and the physician should assure that the billing clerk educates and assists them. Clinical protocols involving nursing personnel can do much to insure that all patients receive needed preventive measures and indicated follow-up.

These aspects of care are ignored in most academic medical centers, both in the care of patients who present themselves for medical services, and in the education of medical students and physicians. In this arena, we have much to learn from the most innovative of our colleagues in community practices.

Physician Assistant Education as a Model for Medical Education

Physician assistant education, probably more by luck than design, fell under the influence of a group of professional educators at an early stage of its development. Having been one of the faculty involved with the first PA program, I can attest that the curriculum for this program was planned exactly like that of the medical school of which it was a part at Duke University. We designed a curriculum along traditional basic science-clinical science lines, and each of the faculty taught what he or she felt the students should learn.

There was no serious thought of the special requirements for training generalists, and there were none among the initial faculty who would have had more than a faint idea of the true nature of a primary care practice. This lack of knowledge of the job which the graduates would be expected to perform did not deter us from trying to cram into the heads of the first classes every bit of information we could, exactly as we did with our medical students.

I can recall the visit of the team that was to provide the first reaccreditation for our program. We fully expected a few compliments and an easy approval. We were amazed to learn that our program did not meet all the requirements, and we were given one year to correct our deficiencies! These deficiencies related to objectives, curricular design, testing and validation of learning and skills, and other details which were very important to the educators but about which we had no knowledge or experience. We quickly learned, with the help of newly hired educators and visits with others, and our one-year provisional approval was converted into a full three-year accreditation.

But we learned more than the requirements. Our students, who were as harassed and anxious as our medical students, were quickly transformed into mature, adult learners who were relaxed and pleased with their learning and who achieved as much or more than they had achieved under the old system. The difference was that they had a defined set of learning and skill-acquisition objectives, and they had a well-designed set of tests to validate their achievements. To our amazement and delight, we had been pushed into an educational design which was much superior to the old one. The new design possessed the following important characteristics:

1. Clear outcome objectives: Prior to the change, we considered that medicine was an impossible field to master, that one could do no better than keep up with rapid advances via constant reading and constant attention to the work of those at the cutting edge. We believed that as much of this new knowledge as possible should be transferred from its source, the medical center, into students' minds to enable them to meet the demands of practice.

We began the new design by selecting the 100 medical diagnoses that brought 98 percent of all patients to primary care practitioners. We then formulated a list of the skills and knowledge required to provide good medical care for these problems. We designed the curriculum to enable students to acquire this information and these skills.

2. *Clear relationship between each lecture and educational exercise and the outcome objectives:* Prior to the change, each lecturer was given a general topic about which he or she had special knowledge and was expected to tell students as much as possible about that topic. The lectures were often filled with the lecturer's own research results, and there was no attempt to confirm that the assigned topic was covered.

The new design provided fewer lectures and more reliance on student reading and self education. We designed each lecture for a particular purpose and provided lecturers with the specific information to be covered, the relationship with the illness or skill to be learned, and the questions the student must be prepared to answer to confirm that the information had been mastered. Those lecturers who did not cover the material assigned were not invited back.

3. *Clear authority and responsibility for curriculum design:* Prior to the change, each disciplinary section of the curriculum was the responsibility of the course director for that discipline. These individuals had total control of the content and the level of the teaching, and the overall program director was only responsible for scheduling, room assignments, and similar tasks.

The new design placed the overall curriculum under the direct authority of the Program Director and a small staff of faculty directly responsible to him. This group had the authority and responsibility for setting learning objectives, breaking them down into lectures and other educational assignments, coordinating various courses, and choosing lecturers and instructors. They controlled the teaching budget and selected those teachers who best performed their jobs, paying the teacher's department for the effort.

4. *Team learning, flexible learning:* A new element introduced with

the new design was team learning. Each class was divided into groups of four, and each group contained students with varied skills and backgrounds. These mixed groups were given time to work together, to search out the information required, and to master the skills expected. The pace of each team was flexible, within broad limits, and the most able were required to help those who were less facile. The result was cooperative and compatible group work, with students bonding together and supporting each other, instead of the highly competitive interaction we are all familiar with among medical students.

Using this new design, the program was able to produce graduates who could move easily into a clinical setting, feel at ease on ward rounds with residents and medical students and perform in a manner that earned respect at all levels, from medical students to attending physicians. They could move easily into positions varying from a specialist's practice to a rural community health center. It was understood that the special procedures and skills required in the new employment, beyond those learned in the program, must be taught by the new practice site and employer, but the employer and the graduate were both confident that a basic set of skills had been acquired.

The above design has kept the overall cost of the PA training program low in comparison to the cost of training medical students. By purchasing teaching time from existing departments, the Duke Physician Assistant Program is able to educate PA students at a cost of about $10,000 per student per year, or $20,000 per student for the entire two-year program. The average cost of educating a medical student in U.S. medical schools is more than $92,000 per student per year, as calculated from data supplied by all schools to the Association of American Medical Colleges for the 1990-91 academic year.[2] This amount may be overstated in that it includes graduate student education and some resident education.

The cost for educating an osteopathic medical student may be a more relevant figure, since osteopathic schools have fewer basic and clinical research functions. The cost of educating each student in these schools is estimated at $45,600 per year, calculated from data supplied by all schools to the Association of Colleges of Osteopathic Medicine for the 1990-91 academic year.[3]

The Duke University program is probably one of the more expensive physician assistant programs, but it produces a very competent generalist practitioner at a cost conservatively estimated at about one-fourth the yearly cost of educating a medical student.[4] Since medical education is four years in length, the total cost of educating a PA is about one-eighth that of a medical student.

U.S. medical schools have much to learn from this experience with physician assistant education. In most medical schools, it would be heresy to suggest that the planning of a medical school curriculum should be removed from the chairs of the basic science and clinical departments, yet this is exactly the lesson which our experience with PA education teaches us. The problem with medical school education is that there is no agreement among the medical school faculty as to what we are training. Each department is attempting to train a clone of its own faculty. Medical students are never told what they are being trained to do, what is expected of them, or what they must learn to meet the demands of their future work.

The PA experiment tells us that we can do a much better job at far less cost by deciding the competencies we wish to attain in medical school education, identifying the knowledge and skills necessary to attain these competencies, and assigning to a small teaching faculty the task of planning the educational experiences of the entire four years of medical school. This group should have the entire teaching budget of the school at its disposal and the authority to purchase required teaching time from faculty in various departments. These faculty members might be primarily engaged and supported by research or clinical activities. I am convinced that we could achieve the same or better results in the education of medical students at a cost comparable with that of the PA student.

Many of our medical schools do not consider the education of medical students as the top priority among the several functions of the medical center. The system of rewards does not favor this function but instead rewards research productivity and, more recently, the performance of highly technical clinical procedures. Is there any incentive to move from the old system to a new one, even if it were shown beyond a shadow of a doubt that the new system was more effective, more efficient, and less expensive?

At this time, there is probably none. But with a new federal administration demanding more care for less money, and with many states pushing for a medical practitioner who is able to meet area needs, we may find that the system of rewards changes rapidly.

In North Carolina, a bill was introduced last year mandating that all medical schools receiving state funds must achieve a 50 percent output of primary care physicians. The bill did not pass, but it will be reintroduced this year. Other states have seen the same type of legislation. State budgets are overburdened, and any system which can do the same job with less money might well be mandated by legislation.

Research funding is already in short supply and is likely to be even tighter. Payment for highly technical procedures may also be sharply curtailed through the Resource-Based Relative Value Scale or price controls. In summary, the incentives are likely to change, and a leaner and more effective educational system may become a high priority. If so, the PA model deserves serious study and a serious trial in the medical school setting.

Finally, educational programs used for the training of midlevel practitioners, particularly PA programs, deserve attention as places to try other educational reforms. The process of education is essentially the same as that involved in education of physicians, but the outcome of the educational process is evident in two years, about one-fourth the time required to produce a medical graduate ready for practice.

An even more useful attribute of these programs is their independence from the dominance and rigidity of the medical school faculty. They are much more open to well-designed educational experiments. The professional educational leadership which has influenced the changes discussed in this paper is still in place in most programs, and this leadership is open to innovation.

For example, the Duke University PA program introduced a system of instruction in the performance of the gynecologic exam utilizing female paid volunteers about 20 years ago. This same system was introduced in the medical student curriculum about 10 years later, having been requested by medical students who had learned of the system from their PA student colleagues. The use of professional actors as instructors in history taking was also introduced by the PA program several years before its introduction in the medical school. In each case, the innovation was well-tested, with good outcome measures, and its introduction in the new setting was consequently much easier.

In summary, PA education has evolved into a remarkably effective and efficient system which could easily be applied in medical student education. If this were done, we could probably produce a better product at about one-fourth the cost. Doing so would require a very different organization of medical student education, placing control in the hands of a very small central teaching faculty, and removing it from traditional departments. PA educational programs could serve as excellent sites for educational innovation.

References

1. Estes EH. The P.A. "experiment" after 25 years: what have we learned? *Federation Bulletin.* 1998;75:259-264.
2. Jolin LD, Jolly P, Krabower JY, Beran R. U.S. medical school finances. *JAMA.* 1992;1149-1155.
3. Association of Colleges of Osteopathic Medicine, Rockville, Md. Personal communication.
4. Carter RD. Director, Physician Assistant Program, Duke University Medical Center, Durham, NC. Personal communication.

9

Government Health Policy and the Non-Physician Practitioner: A Closer Look

Henry Desmarais

N ON-PHYSICIAN PRACTITIONERS, INCLUDING PHYSI-cian assistants (PAs) and nurse practitioners (NPs), play an increasingly important role in providing primary care and other health services in the United States. The federal and state governments play a critical role in determining the types of services these practitioners may provide, the circumstances under which they may be provided, and the rules of reimbursement. Government policies have evolved over time and are far from uniform or stable. Moreover, they have been influenced by concerns about health care access problems, the views of other practitioners — especially physicians — fiscal considerations, and a variety of other factors. Also important have been studies suggesting that the quality of care provided by non-physician practitioners "is equivalent to the quality of comparable services provided by physicians"[1] and that these practitioners can successfully substitute for physicians in providing the bulk of care provided in outpatient primary care settings.[2]

Currently, heightened concerns about health care coverage gaps and the costs of care and growing prospects for comprehensive reform of the U.S. health care financing and delivery systems provide opportune circumstances to examine the trends and driving forces in federal and state policies regarding reimbursement and scope of practice of non-physician primary care providers. This paper will discuss these issues, concentrating on physician assistants and, to a somewhat lesser extent, nurse practitioners.

Coverage of Services

Services provided by PAs, NPs, and a variety of other non-physicians are covered under Medicare, Medicaid, and other public and private health benefit programs. Coverage is generally dependent upon the site of service, the practitioner's relationship with a supervising or collaborating physician, the applicable scope-of-practice act, and other factors. Some states even mandate that all health insurance policies sold within their borders cover services provided by these non-physician practitioners (mandated inclusion), provide an option for such coverage (mandated offering), or at least not discriminate in the treatment of certain practitioners with respect to coverage of, or payment for, their services.

Under Medicare, coverage for the services of PAs and NPs has improved over time. From the beginning of the program, services of these practitioners could be covered as "incident to" physicians' services. In other words, under this provision, the "services of nurses and other assistants that are commonly furnished as a necessary adjunct to the physician's in-office service" are covered as physicians' services, unless the services in question "traditionally have been reserved to physicians."[3] In effect, under the "incident to" provision, services provided by non-physicians are covered — and paid for — as if they were provided by the physician. In fact, program administrators often have no easy way of knowing whether a service was provided by a physician or by someone employed by the physician.

Recently, Medicare has explicitly provided separate coverage for at least some of the services provided by PAs and NPs. The following services are now covered for both provider groups: rural health clinic services, services to homebound patients in areas without a home health agency, and services in managed care organizations having a risk-based contract with the Medicare program, under which payment is made on a capitated, rather than fee-for-service, basis.

In addition, Medicare covers services provided by PAs in rural health professional shortage areas and services provided by NPs in all rural areas. Medicare specifically covers PA services performed in urban and rural hospitals and nursing facilities, and PAs serving as assistants at surgery, if such services would be covered if performed by a physician. In the case of NPs, coverage on a fee-for-service basis outside of rural areas is specifically available only for services performed in nursing facilities. Finally, Medicare coverage rules specify that PAs must be under the supervision of a physician and that NPs must be working in collaboration with a physician.

With respect to Medicaid, states *must* cover NP and PA services provided in rural health clinics. No other federal mandates apply to PA services. However, states are *required* to include the services of certified pediatric and family nurse practitioners in their Medicaid benefit package, effective July 1, 1990.[4] States may also provide broader coverage of PA and NP services, and many have availed themselves of this option. In fact, generally speaking, Medicaid policies are less restrictive than comparable Medicare rules in that they tend not to restrict coverage to particular sites of care or provide preferential treatment of services performed in rural, as opposed to urban settings.

Two states — Montana and South Dakota — even allow PAs to bill directly for services provided to Medicaid patients.[5] However, some Medicaid programs still do not cover all the services which PAs and NPs are capable of performing under their respective scope-of-practice acts. In addition, some states still do not cover the services of NPs under Medicaid because their scope-of-practice acts do not distinguish between registered nurses generally and those with advanced training, such as NPs.[6]

A December 1992 report by the Blue Cross and Blue Shield Association notes that, with respect to private health insurance policies, 17 states mandate services provided by NPs (two of which involve mandated offering) and three states (Maryland, Michigan, and Montana) mandate the inclusion of physician assistants' services.[7] Such state mandates do not affect self-insured organizations, including many large employers, whose benefit, coverage and payment decisions are shielded by provisions of the Employee Retirement Income Security Act.

Payment

Payment for the services of PAs and NPs is generally based on payment amounts for the same or similar services provided by physicians, with payment often set at some percentage (usually less than 100 percent) of the amount that would be paid if the service were performed by a physician. The applicable percentage may vary depending upon the site of service. PAs and NPs may even be paid different amounts for the same service. For example, Medicare currently pays PAs as follows:

- For services performed in a hospital setting (other than as an assistant at surgery), payment may not exceed 75 percent of the amount that Medicare would pay if the service were performed by a physician.
- For assistant at surgery services, payment may not exceed 65 percent of the amount that would be paid a physician.
- For services provided in a nursing facility, payment may not exceed 85 percent of the amount that would be paid a physician.
- For all other covered services *performed in a rural health professional shortage area,* payment may not exceed 85 percent of the amount that would be paid a physician.

In the case of NPs, Medicare will pay no more than 75 percent of the physician fee for hospital services (including assistance at surgery) provided in rural areas and no more than 85 percent of the physician fee for all other services performed in these areas, as well as for services provided in urban nursing facilities.

With respect to Medicaid, states have considerable discretion in setting payment rates for services provided by NPs and PAs. Some Medicaid programs (and some other third-party payers as well) pay both physicians and non-physicians the same rate, but this practice is more likely where payment amounts are low.

In the case of PAs, Medicare payments always are made to the PA's employer (e.g., the physician, the managed care organization, or the rural health clinic). In contrast, NPs may bill Medicare in their own right for covered services provided in rural settings. In addition, certified pediatric and family nurse practitioners may receive direct payment for services covered under Medicaid if they so choose. States also have the option of paying all NPs directly if they elect to cover such services under their respective Medicaid programs.

Payment for PA and NP services is further complicated by the fact that, under Medicare's "incident to" rules, a service provided by a PA or NP is paid as if it were performed by a physician — i.e., at 100 percent of the physician fee schedule amount. Of course, in such cases, the physician is presumably providing direct (on-site) supervision. Obviously, physician employers of PAs and NPs have a financial incentive to bill for the services of PA and NP employees under this "incident to" policy, whenever possible, in order to receive 100 percent of the applicable physician fee rather than some lesser amount.

Finally, current Medicare rules preclude asking patients to pay out-of-pocket more than the applicable coinsurance and deductible amounts for covered NP and PA services.

Scope of Practice

Scope of practice for PAs and NPs — and other health care practitioners as well — is a state prerogative. For this reason, it varies considerably across the country.

Key scope-of-practice issues include: the degree of specificity in designating permitted services, the nature of any required physician supervisory or collaborative role, and the circumstances under which an NP or PA may prescribe medications, if at all. With respect to services, the Alabama scope-of-practice act for PAs specifically proscribes lumbar punctures, thoracentesis, joint aspiration, and other procedures. Other states — for example, Florida — specify that certain procedures, such as the insertion of chest tubes, may be performed, but only when the supervising physician is on the premises. In other locales, such as Kansas, the scope of practice includes "[d]elegated acts constituting the practice of medicine and surgery that can be competently performed by the PA, based on his or her education, skill, and experience."[8]

Scope-of-practice acts for PAs and NPs also vary with respect to required physician supervision, although most states do not require direct (on-site) supervision by physicians.[9] For example, in the case of PAs, the District of Columbia specifies that the supervising physician must be within a 15-mile radius of the city and available in person or by communication device. Maryland expects the physician to exercise on-site supervision or immediately available direction. In Virginia, the level of required physician supervision for PAs is determined on an individual basis by the State Board of Medicine, and chart review by the physician is required within 24 hours. In Louisiana, the PA may not work when the supervising physician is absent or off duty unless the physician can be physically present within 30 minutes.

With respect to the prescribing and dispensing of drugs, PA and

NP scope-of-practice acts vary enormously. About 34 states and the District of Columbia provide PAs with some prescriptive authority. Some states allow PAs to prescribe only non-controlled substances or only drugs listed on an approved formulary. Other states allow PAs to prescribe certain classes of controlled substances as well as non-controlled drugs.

Health System Reform

While reform of the U.S. health care financing and delivery system might once have been primarily motivated by concerns about health coverage gaps, health care cost containment now appears to have taken a central place in the debate. Relatively ill-defined terms like "managed competition" and "global budgets" are touted by some as the answers to burgeoning health care costs. Others advocate adoption of a single-payer or all-payer system, under which the federal government would either pay for all the care, or be responsible for setting maximum payment rates for all third-party payers.

Health care cost containment fervor could further increase the demand for non-physician providers. This increase would be particularly likely if payment for health care services under any reform plan became increasingly or primarily based on per-capita or other bundled arrangements, rather than the more traditional fee-for-service policies. Capitated or bundled payment approaches provide tremendous financial incentives for delivering services in the most cost-effective manner possible (e.g., using the least costly health care personnel qualified to provide them). However, other outcomes are also possible, especially as the supply of physicians increases or if controls of some kind are imposed to reduce the utilization of — or patient demand for — health care services or limit patient choice of provider.

Roles and Distribution of Non-Physician Personnel

There is considerable concern about the shortage of primary care providers, especially in health professional shortage areas. The Graduate Medical Education National Advisory Committee and many other entities have recommended steps to address this problem.[10] Curiously, the current federal criteria for designating primary care health professional shortage areas do not take into account the availability of non-physician personnel, such as nurse practitioners, physician assistants, and certified nurse midwives, who certainly are qualified to provide the bulk of primary care services.

In fact, one could argue that there really has not been any systematic discussion about the appropriate roles of various physician and non-physician health care personnel in providing primary care services or health care services generally. Such a discussion will likely become more important over time, especially as the supply of physicians increases, since there is always the potential for unproductive competition between physicians and non-physicians in delivery of services that both groups are qualified to provide, or even for anti-competitive actions to be taken by one group against another. As an example of the tension that can be created between different types of practitioners, the American Medical Association has opposed permitting NPs to write prescriptions without physician supervision.[11]

Since the resources involved in training physicians are much greater than those required to train non-physician health care personnel, and since the payments for services provided by the former are generally greater than those when the same services are provided by the latter, it would appear to be in society's best interest to determine the most efficient and effective use of different types of health care personnel.

Interestingly, while many PAs and NPs originally chose primary care practice in rural areas, there now appears to be a shift toward specialty practice in urban areas. For example, from 1978 to 1989, the number of PAs employed in primary care specialties actually declined between 1 and 2 percent per year. Similarly, while 27 percent of PAs were working in towns of less than 10,000 in 1981, only 15.4 percent of PAs were doing so in 1991. This shift appears to be due, at least in part, to the increased demand for PAs by urban employers and by higher paying non-primary care physicians.[12]

Differential Treatment of Providers

State and federal policies distinguish between PAs and NPs and in some cases even between different NP specialties, sometimes for unexplained reasons. For example, it is not intuitively obvious why Medicare should cover NP services in all settings in all rural areas but only provide equivalent coverage for PA services performed in rural locales designated as health professional shortage areas. It is also not clear why Medicare should pay NPs more than PAs for assistance at surgery in rural areas or pay only PAs for assistance at surgery in urban areas.

In addition, serious questions have been raised about the appropriateness of current Medicaid policies that mandate direct reimbursement of only some NP specialties, prompting at least one legislative proposal to expand the mandate to cover all NPs and clinical nurse specialists as well.[13] Medicare's method for reimbursing hospitals for indirect medical education costs is considered yet another example of a problematic, differential payment policy. In this case, the payment formulae account for the number of residents in a graduate medical education program but not the PAs increasingly being hired to substitute for these residents, even though the PA employment costs in these positions are believed to "roughly approximate those of physician residents."[14]

Policy makers should determine whether such differential policies are justified or whether they simply pose undue barriers to the most efficient and effective use of these non-physician primary care providers.

In a similar vein, considerable variation in state scope-of-practice acts for non-physician primary care providers means there is considerable variation in the roles these providers can play across the country. For example, there is evidence that more liberal prescriptive authority for PAs is associated with a higher proportion of PAs working in rural areas.[15] While imputing a causal link between these two variables would be inappropriate, there is no doubt that PAs and NPs with little or no prescriptive authority must play a different role than those with greater authority to prescribe and dispense controlled and non-controlled substances.

There also continues to be some discussion about reimbursement policies relating to services provided by PAs and NPs. The Physician Payment Review Commission believes that, at least under the Medicare program, these non-physician practitioners should "continue to have payments that differ from those of physicians...adjusted to reflect differences in the investments in education and training between each NPP [non-physician practitioner] category and physicians [and the] significantly lower malpractice expenses" of PAs and NPs.[16] The Commission also recommended that such services be clearly identified on claim forms, but the Health Care Financing Administration ultimately decided not to adopt such a requirement, at least for the time being, because of concerns raised by others about associated administrative and paperwork burdens.[17]

A 1991 survey by the Blue Cross and Blue Shield Association found that "just over half the plans across the country reimburse NPs and PAs for treating patients, and two-thirds of these said they pay PAs and NPs the *same* fees they do MDs for the same services" [emphasis added].[18] In fact, many have advocated that both physicians and non-physicians should receive "equal pay for equal work." However, it has been difficult to establish — in a manner convincing to all affected parties — the circumstances under which a service can be considered "the same" whether provided by a physician or a non-physician practitioner.

As noted above, even Medicare's own rules are confusing on this point, since the program will pay 100 percent of the physician fee schedule amount for PA or NP services provided "incident to" a physician's service but a lower percentage for other PA and NP services. Moreover, at least some of the provisions expanding coverage for PA and NP services were advocated on the basis of cost-effectiveness, i.e., that these services would substitute for more expensive physicians' services. Budget estimators, however, have traditionally assumed that expanded coverage for PA and NP services would increase aggregate spending, since more services would be provided overall.

Future Evolution of NP and PA Programs

Finally, at a time when many are seeking every way possible to make the U.S. health care system more efficient and effective, it might be fruitful to consider whether the current separate and distinct natures of NP and PA training programs remain appropriate, or whether both types of programs might benefit by borrowing from one another. Certainly, the current programs are often distinguished by whether they are governed by the "nursing model" or the "medical model," but the practitioners prepared by these different training programs are frequently considered interchangeable.

It might, therefore, be useful to examine whether both types of programs should evolve in one direction. In addition, given current and anticipated health care needs as well as the overall economic and policy environment, it would seem appropriate to discuss whether current distinctions in the training, licensing, utilization, and payment of NPs and PAs are likely to make sense over the longer term.

References

1. United States Congress, Office of Technology Assessment. *Nurse Practitioners, Physician Assistants, and Certified Nurse-Midwives: A Policy Analysis.* Washington, DC: Government Printing Office; 1986.
2. Hooker RS, Freeborn DK. The utilization of physician assistants in a managed health care system. *Public Health Reports.* 1991;106:90-94.
3. Health Care Financing Administration. *Medicare Carriers Manual,* section 2050.3. Baltimore, Md: Health Care Financing Administration.
4. U.S. House of Representatives, Committee on Energy and Commerce. *Medicaid Source Book: Background Data and Analysis (A 1993 Update).* Washington, DC: Government Printing Office; 1993.
5. Physician Payment Review Commission. *Annual Report to Congress.* Washington, DC: Physician Payment Review Commission; 1993.
6. Physician Payment Review Commission. *Annual Report to Congress.* 1993.
7. Laudicina SS, *Impact of State Basic Benefit Laws on the Uninsured.* Washington, DC: Blue Cross Blue Shield Association; December 1992.
8. American Academy of Physician Assistants. *State Laws for Physician Assistants.* Alexandria, Va: American Academy of Physician Assistants; December 1992.
9. Physician Payment Review Commission. *Annual Report to Congress. 1993.*
10. For example, see Council on Graduate Medical Education. *Improving Access to Health Care Through Physician Workforce Reform: Directions for the 21st Century.* Washington, DC: United States Department of Health and Human Services; 1992.
11. Gesensway D. Despite medicine's protests, NPs and PAs winning turf as primary care practitioners. *ACP Observer.* December 1992:12.
12. U.S. Department of Health and Human Services. *Health Personnel in the United States, Eighth Report to Congress, 1991.* Washington, DC: Government Printing Office; 1992.
13. U.S. Congress. *Medicaid Nursing Incentive Act of 1993.* S. 466, 103rd Congress, 1st Session; 1993.
14. Cawley JF. Physician assistants: whither their roles in primary care? Presentation to the Third Annual Primary Care Research Conference, Agency for Health Care Policy and Research; January 12, 1993; Atlanta, Ga.
15. Willis J. Is the PA supply in rural America dwindling? *J Am Acad Physician Assistants.* 1990;3:433-5.
16. Physician Payment Review Commission. *Annual Report to Congress.* Washington, DC: Physician Payment Review Commission; 1991.
17. U.S. General Services Administration. *Federal Register.* 1991;56(227):59604-5.
18. Gesensway D. Despite medicine's protests. *ACP Observer.* December 1992:12.

OREGON HEALTH SCIENCES UNIVERSITY
PHYSICIAN ASSISTANT PROGRAM
GH219
3181 SW SAM JACKSON PARK RD
PORTLAND OR 97201